# María José Ortiz Sainz de Rozas

## Efficacy of hyperbaric oxygen therapy

María José Ortiz Sainz de Rozas

# Efficacy of hyperbaric oxygen therapy

## in the rescue treatment of idiopathic sudden sudden hearing loss

ScienciaScripts

**Imprint**

Any brand names and product names mentioned in this book are subject to trademark, brand or patent protection and are trademarks or registered trademarks of their respective holders. The use of brand names, product names, common names, trade names, product descriptions etc. even without a particular marking in this work is in no way to be construed to mean that such names may be regarded as unrestricted in respect of trademark and brand protection legislation and could thus be used by anyone.

Cover image: www.ingimage.com

This book is a translation from the original published under ISBN 978-613-9-41175-7.

Publisher:
Sciencia Scripts
is a trademark of
Dodo Books Indian Ocean Ltd. and OmniScriptum S.R.L publishing group

120 High Road, East Finchley, London, N2 9ED, United Kingdom
Str. Armeneasca 28/1, office 1, Chisinau MD-2012, Republic of Moldova, Europe
Printed at: see last page
**ISBN: 978-620-8-26710-0**

**DEDICATIONS**

*To my mother, brothers and Guillermo for supporting me and loving me unconditionally, for always believing in me and not letting me give up.*

# ACKNOWLEDGEMENTS

*To my parents for giving me all the tools to achieve my goals.*
*To my teachers for all their teachings and experiences.*
*To the UAS, the Civil Hospital of Culiacán and CIDOCS for the opportunity they have given me to be able to my speciality.*
*To CONACYT for the support given during my residency.*

## TABLE OF CONTENTS

# I SUMMARY

***Introduction:** Sudden idiopathic hearing loss is a common ENT emergency of unknown aetiology and pathogenesis; for its rescue treatment, corticosteroids are the most accepted drugs, however, hyperbaric oxygen therapy, intended to contribute to the delivery of positive pressure to the inner ear vasculature and oxygen to the tissues, has been implemented as an adjunctive therapy to intratympanic steroid application or as an isolated rescue therapy.*

***Objective(s):** To evaluate the efficacy and hearing outcomes of hyperbaric oxygen therapy as a rescue treatment for idiopathic sudden sudden hearing loss. To determine the degree of hearing recovery and improvement.*

***Material and methods:** Retrospective study, from March 2021 to September 2023. Patients diagnosed with idiopathic sudden sudden hearing loss who received hyperbaric oxygen therapy as rescue treatment were included. Demographic aspects of the patients, time of evolution and PTA (average of pure tones) at diagnosis, pre and post hyperbaric chamber will be analysed.*

***Results:** Thirty-eight patients were recruited, ranging in age from 26 to 75 years (mean 51.4 years), 60.5% female and 39% male. The pre-hyperbaric chamber PTA was 63.4 dB, and post-hyperbaric chamber 48.1 dB; with an overall hearing gain of 15 dB (p= 0.000). 26.3% of the patients had complete recovery, 36.8% had moderate recovery, the remaining 36.8% had poor recovery.*

***Conclusion.** Hyperbaric oxygen therapy is a therapy that benefits hearing in patients with idiopathic sudden sudden hearing loss, especially when added to other systemic transthympanic therapies, with the greatest benefit during the first 4 weeks after onset.*

***Keywords:** idiopathic sudden sudden hearing loss, hyperbaric chamber, rescue treatment.*

## II THEORETICAL FRAMEWORK

**History**

Idiopathic sudden hearing loss is an otological condition described by the patient as frightening and distressing, developing within seventy-two hours, most commonly overnight upon awakening, with a hearing loss of more than 30 dB in at least 3 consecutive frequencies in the audiological record. Because of its suddenness, it requires prompt attention and is classified as an emergency for the specialised otorhinolaryngologist.[1]

**Epidemiology**

Worldwide, there are an estimated 466 million hearing impaired people, of which 34 million are paediatric, according to the latest data reported by the World Health Organization.[2]

Idiopathic sudden hearing loss is a frequent otological emergency. It accounts for 2-3% of the otolaryngology specialist's daily consultation. Its incidence is approximately 5-20 persons per 100,000 annually in the United States, with a total of 66,000 cases each year. The incidence figure can be as high as 160 cases per 100,000 per year, reported in Germany.[3]

It has a peak incidence at 60 years of age, an age range of 50-60 years, with equal distribution between the sexes. It most often presents unilaterally, but bilateral involvement may occur in 1-5% of patients.[4]

It may present as an isolated clinical process or in combination with an underlying disease, where its behaviour is identified as a hearing loss of unknown origin and one as SSNHL itself.[5.]

It generates a potential risk of accidents in daily life activities such as crossing streets or socialising, by drastically reducing the risk of accidents. sensory organ, unilaterally or bilaterally, essential for spatial perception and sound source localisation, as well as increasing the likelihood of long- and short-term disability.[1]

Dizziness occurs in 30-60% of cases. Its clinical presentation, together with vertigo (20-57%), means a worse prognosis. Tinnitus is constant, occurring in 70% of cases. It may persist in those with spontaneous or self-limited improvement or be part of the patient's initial complaint in the emergency department or outpatient clinic, generating a new public health problem due to its psychological involvement and the patient's quality of life, which may even be classified in the long term as a co-morbidity. Therefore, clinical presentation with any of these three symptoms has a major impact on quality of life. [1,4]

In addition to this, there are higher health and individual costs for patients in terms of audiological follow-up, long- and short-term treatment techniques with uncertain effectiveness and the exclusion of secondary pathologies, especially neoplastic ones with ancillary imaging and laboratory studies, as well as adequate rehabilitation after the crucial two-week period following the onset of symptoms, such as hearing aids or implantable hearing devices. Despite the health and public health burden involved, it is also important to highlight the possibility of spontaneous recovery in up to 45-65%, by way of contrast, poor recovery is possible with timely treatment and diagnosis that ends up leaving the patient with permanent hearing loss, persistent tinnitus and an evident reduction in quality of life. [5]

**Aetiology**


For the most part, the specific cause is unknown and it is classified as idiopathic in origin, however, secondary causes have been proposed that should be evaluated in the first instance before it is treated as an otological condition of unknown cause.

It remains controversial both in terms of pathophysiology and aetiology. It is attributed to be 90% idiopathic in origin, where throughout history it has been attempted to provide an objective explanation for the underlying mechanism. The remaining 10% are considered to be secondary causes. [6]

Among the secondary aetiological causes to be ruled out are viral infectious diseases: rubella, measles, mumps, herpes simplex virus, HIV, infectious mononucleosis due to cytomegalovirus or Epstein Barr virus and their associated opportunistic diseases. Bacterial infectious pathology such as Lyme disease, syphilis, meningitis; Neoplastic causes with involvement of the pontocerebellar angle or the internal auditory canal such as: vestibular schwannoma, cholesteatoma, cholesterol granuloma, meningiomas, among others; Traumatic causes such as after suffering a cranioencephalic trauma or having generated a post-infectious perilymphatic fistula. [7]

It is also essential to rule out diseases that may suddenly debut with unilateral or bilateral hypoacusis, such as Meniere's disease, multiple sclerosis, Cogan's syndrome, migraine, polyarteritis nodosa, temporal artery arteritis or systemic lupus erythematosus, thromboangiitis obliterans (Buerger's disease), angiopathies developed in patients with diabetes mellitus, macroglobulinemias or sickle cell anaemia. As well as the use of drugs with potential otological damage, including in spinal anaesthesia, which has been associated with up to 40%. [4,7]

**Pathophysiology and histology**

The mechanisms by which the inner ear is damaged and idiopathic sudden hypoacusis is generated have been proposed over time, without finding a definitive cause after having excluded secondary aetiologies and defining a purely idiopathic condition. Among them, inflammatory processes following viral infections of probable subclinical evolution and with cochlear invasion, latent viral reactivation in the cochlear spiral ganglion stand out. [4,7]

Probable autoimmune mechanisms following systemic infection are: alterations in the haemodynamics and vasculature of the inner ear; hypercoagulability documented in patients who develop idiopathic sudden hypoacusis; or cochlear ischaemia, due to the particularity of the inner ear circulation of not having collateral circulation; as well as decreased oxygen pressure with consequent hypoxia. [4,7,8, 9]

The cochlear vasculature is particularly susceptible to changes in blood supply, the blood supply being provided by the labyrinthine artery, with no collateral vascular supply. It can be altered by vasospasm and any other cause that alters the blood supply, by the occlusive or partially occlusive presence of the vessel due to vasospasm, thrombi or emboli. Damage at this level correlates with the sudden evolution characteristic of idiopathic sudden hearing loss and makes it an important mechanism of inner ear injury, on which treatment has historically been based. However, cardiovascular risk factors, hypercholesterolemia and diabetes mellitus remain a likely pathophysiological explanation. [4,7,8, 9]

Histological evidence has been documented in human and animal temporal bones, with disruption of labyrinthine vessels and intralabyrinthine haemorrhage, with consequent fibrosis and cochlear ossification. [4]

The viral infectious aetiology has been controversial due to the presence of viral pictures of upper respiratory tract referenced days prior to the development of sudden hypoacusis. In addition, seroconversion for multiple viral aetiologies has been documented in patients who develop idiopathic sudden hypoacusis and in the histopathology of temporal bones, lesions coinciding with viral aetiologies: atrophy of the tectorial membrane and stria vascularis, loss of hair cells and of the cochlear nervous component.[7] Another probable pathophysiological mechanism of idiopathic sudden hypoacusis has been proposed as the rupture of intracochlear membranes, from those that are responsible for making an anatomical separation between the inner ear and the middle ear, or those that structure the inner part of the cochlea and separate the endolymph from the perilymph. When one or both of these membranes rupture, there is a mixing of intracochlear fluids, a decrease in endocochlear potential, and the physiological and anatomical pathway through which sound travels is disrupted. Leakage of perilymph into the middle ear through the oval window or through the round window has been proposed to subsequently cause a pathophysiological state of relative endolymphatic hydrops, all as part of a process leading to a clinical end of sensorineural hearing loss reported by the patient and subsequently documented by audiometry.[10]

**Diagnosis**

To begin with the appropriate approach, a complete clinical history is required to rule out autoimmune, chronic degenerative, vascular, infectious, neurological and neurological risk comorbidities and the use of ototoxic drugs. The clinical course of the disease and the evolution of the hypoacusis should be investigated, ruling out any other associated risk symptoms that indicate the probable aetiology of an identifiable or organic cause of idiopathic sudden hypoacusis: neurological focality (diplopia, dysarthria, headache, ataxia, confusion, altered mental status, focal facial or body weakness), bilateral vestibular symptomatology, oscillopsia, spontaneous or gaze-evoked or downbeat nystagmus, signs of lacrimation, ocular pain, redness or photophobia, recent acoustic trauma, head trauma, barotrauma, fluctuating hearing loss or sudden bilateral hearing loss. [1,7, 10]

Audiometry is the basic and obligatory technique for diagnosing idiopathic sudden sudden hearing loss. Above all to rule out conductive hearing loss and to confirm the typical pattern of three consecutive frequencies and a loss of more than 30 dB of sensorineural characteristics. This is a key point that defines the subsequent management of the patient and requires promptness within 14 days after the onset of symptoms.
Normal hearing prior to the onset of hearing loss or symmetrical bilateral hearing loss is taken as a reference. Hearing loss is usually defined by comparing hearing between the two ears. According to the American National Standards Institute, both diagnostic and follow-up

evaluations should have an initial otoscopy, obtain correct masking and hearing thresholds at frequencies of 250-8000 Hz, assessment of speech frequencies with associated pure tone averaging (PTA) and speech recognition testing (WSR) with calculation of the percentage of correct responses to predict probable unobvious asymmetry during pure tone audiometry. [1,4,7,10]Other techniques that complete the comprehensive study of idiopathic sudden hearing loss are acoustic immittance measurements, which are useful for ruling out conductive hearing loss. In addition to the above, the stapedial acoustic reflex, otoacoustic emissions (OAE), the functionality and preservation of the outer hair cells are reserved in the absence of additional methods available for diagnosis and discriminate between hearing loss of sensory or neural origin, however, they remain additional studies that lack specificity when performed individually, require association and audiometric confirmation.[11]

In order to rule out aetiologies before classifying the clinical picture as idiopathic, the most frequent aetiology of idiopathic sudden hypoacusis, auxiliary laboratory studies are used, such as: complete blood count, to rule out polycythaemia, thrombosis, leukaemia or anaemia; erythrocyte sedimentation rate, 68 kD test and/or antinuclear antibodies (ANA), for autoimmune pathology; FTA-ABS, VDRL, HIV ELISA, for retrovirus or Treponema Pallidum infectious pathologies; prothrombin time and activated partial thromboplastin time with INR, for history of coagulopathies; thyroid function tests, to rule out hypothyroidism, as another possible cause.[1]

It is essential to use magnetic resonance imaging of the skull with gadolinium to evaluate structures of the internal auditory canal, inner ear, brainstem and pontocerebellar angle. It should be performed in all patients presenting to the emergency department or outpatient clinic with a pattern of unilateral hearing loss of recent onset, sudden course, due to the high risk of retrocochlear neoplastic pathology. The most characteristic entity is vestibular schwannoma, a pathology that can be treated in a timely manner when detected in early stages, by means of the Gold Standard for its diagnosis, which is magnetic resonance imaging with a protocol of modalities: CISS or FIESTA and contrasted T1. Among other neoplastic pathologies, it stands out for having an initial clinical course similar to idiopathic sudden hypoacusis, in 10.2%. Its prevalence in patients with sudden hearing loss is not negligible and ranges from 0.8% to 3%. MRI may also find evidence of multiple sclerosis or cochlear inflammation.[12]ABR, used for the diagnostic approach to retrocochlear pathology, is not very sensitive; it requires confirmation by imaging techniques after providing a result coincident with retrocochlear pathology, prolongation of wave V. Its limitations are that it can miss intracanalicular (vestibular schwannoma) in up to 42%; its sensitivity is linked toproportionally to the degree of hearing loss and, in patients with mild hearing loss, there are more false negatives from the test. Likewise, results suggestive of retrocochlear pathology will only appear when the tumours of the cerebellopontine angle are larger than 1 cm. Its application is contraindicated when the hearing loss is greater than 80 dB at 4,000 Hz. Therefore, if the result is normal, the pathology is not completely ruled out and a six-month audiological follow-up is required. Its use is reserved for patients who cannot undergo MRI.[13]

Cranial computed tomography, however, is of little importance for the diagnosis of idiopathic sudden hearing loss. Its usual slices are 0.5 mm, which are not specific to basic anatomical areas intended to be evaluated in detail such as the internal auditory canal, and its daily use is aimed at, and justified in cases where there is a high suspicion of ischaemic or haemorrhagic stroke, who are accompanied by a clinical presentation of neurological focality, refer previous cranioencephalic trauma, claustrophobia, suspicion of an immersed lesion in the temporal bone or cholesteatomatous disease. [1,7]

According to the American College of Radiology (ACR) for sudden idiopathic hypoacusis, the use of tomography is evaluated at number "3", for its level of evidence in itself is an appropriate imaging study for diagnosis, this level expresses that cranial tomography is a study that is not very useful in diagnosis; it has its exceptions when the patients have specific specifications that merit its use. On the other hand, it is subject to a risk greater than the benefit obtained as a final result, such as renal damage or anaphylaxis associated with the application of intravenous contrast medium or exposure to radiation.[14]


**Treatment**


In the past, based on pathophysiological theories: rupture of intracochlear membranes, occlusion or vascular pathology, infectious or autoimmune processes, the following drugs were used as alternative therapies and are still optional therapies: antivirals, vasodilators, thrombolytics and vasoactive agents. These are optional therapies that do not have shown sufficient effectiveness to be used routinely and, in contrast, may be associated with adverse effects.Currently, corticosteroids, the most accepted and effective drugs, are available for treatment, their use in daily clinical practice as a cornerstone for both immediate treatment, during the first two weeks of symptomatology onset, as well as rescue treatment after two to six weeks of symptom onset. Its route of administration is systemic, oral or intravenous or intratympanic, with different mechanisms of action and indications for different types of patients, either alone or in combination with other therapies. Treatment will always be individualised for each case.[15]

While steroid therapy has been reported to be highly effective, a small percentage may not document any improvement and may benefit from salvage therapy.

Initial treatment with corticosteroids is the most indicated management. It is recommended to start within the first two weeks of the onset of symptomatology. Its mechanism of action lies in the fact that it is possible to stop the cell death cascade, cause a reversal or stop the apoptotic pathways in the injured cochlear hair cells and associated inflammation that leads to the pathophysiology of idiopathic sudden hearing loss. Prednisolone, prednisone, dexamethasone, methylprednisolone and prednisolone have been discussed for use via the intratympanic or systemic route, where they have been compared in several randomised clinical trials with evidence of a clear significant difference in the effectiveness of one or the other route of administration, and even the same hearing recovery has been seen between the two. The largest comparative study of these two therapies as initial management did not identify substantially different or comparative improvement in hearing when using either intratympanic methylprednisolone at a concentration of 40 mg/ml or oral prednisone at a ceiling dose of 60 mg per day for 14 days. Combined, systemic intratympanic therapy has also been effective and has been extensively studied in multiple reviews, with 20 dB improvements in PTA and 30% improvements in voice discrimination[15] ; however, it remains a matter of debate as to whether this recovery over the period of crucial two-week window, it is possible that this is also a "false improvement" because of the possibility of spontaneous recovery.[15]

As explained in previous paragraphs, the benefits of any therapy in general, but in this case corticosteroid therapy because it is the most widely accepted, are greater when used within the 15-day window following the onset of the condition, as well as the probable spontaneous recovery without medical intervention of any kind. Recovery may also occur later in a smaller percentage, very similar to what happens with corticosteroid therapy, which decreases in benefit when used between the fourth and sixth week.

The recommended prednisone regimen is at a dose of 1mg/kg/day with a maximum dose of 60 mg/day, a methylprednisolone equivalent of 48 mg and dexamethasone of 10 mg. An initial maximum dose for four days with dose reduction every other day for the next 10 days, or maximum dose for 7 to 10 days with dose reduction for one week, or a third option is to provide therapy for 4 weeks of maximum dose with dose reduction every other day thereafter. Notable adverse effects include: uncontrolled diabetes mellitus, susceptibility to infection, gastric irritation, nervousness, osteoporosis, fluid retention, facial oedema, increased appetite, muscle weakness, insomnia, glaucoma, cataracts, blurred vision and weight gain. All of which tend to occur with prolonged, chronic use. Despite this, its use remains risky in: uncontrolled diabetes mellitus, hypertension, peptic acid disease, glaucoma, tuberculosis, with psychiatric reaction to corticosteroids, the recommendation of therapy is maintained, but by intratympanic route, to avoid the burden of damage to the quality of life and hearing impairment that can generate idiopathic sudden hypoacusis in the long term.[16]

The intratympanic route of administration is reserved for the patients described in the previous paragraph. When applied in this way, it is possible to achieve high perilymphatic concentrations of the medicinal product and to enhance the local use of the medicinal product. Methylprednisolone and dexamethasone, at concentrations of >30 mg/dl and 4-24 mg/dl respectively, are available for use; they are administered for 15-30 minutes in the affected ear, with a frequency of once daily or once weekly. Possible adverse effects are: pain, infection, dizziness with possible vasovagal process or episode of syncope or persistent tympanic perforation.[17]

Another form of corticosteroid use is salvage therapy, which is performed after documented failure of hearing recovery following initial therapy of any kind (HBOT, systemic or topical steroids, or simply observation). Intratympanic use is preferred. In general, there is no specific evidence to indicate when it is advisable to start treatment or how often it should be applied. It is applied on a step-by-step basis, commonly used during the 2 to 7 days following the end of systemic steroid therapy, by means of intra-tympanic injections or myringotomy with tympanostomy tubes. Some options are the use of dexamethasone at a dose of 4-5 mg/ml for 2-6 injections within 2 weeks, 2-7 days after completion of systemic steroid therapy or the use of methylprednisolone 40 mg in 1 ml of sodium bicarbonate injections every 3 days or daily to complete 4 doses, within 7 days of completion of systemic therapy or a variable time as deemed appropriate by the clinician.[18]

On the other hand, hyperbaric oxygen therapy (HBO) was first used as a treatment option for idiopathic sudden sudden hearing loss in 1970, but had previously been tested in 1960 as an adjunctive treatment for sudden hearing loss in Germany and France. It was approved for the treatment of this entity in October 2011 by the Underseas and Hyperbaric Medical Society

(UHMS).[19]The main reason for using it in the treatment of idiopathic sudden hypoacusis is after having had the physiopathological suspicion of hypoxia at the level of the inner ear tissues. Its benefits are haemodynamic by increasing oxygen pressure and its delivery to the cochlear tissue, a structure sensitive to ischaemia, immunological and the reduction of oedema and tissue hypoxia. Its therapeutic use lies in providing high-pressure oxygenation to the inner ear and restoring hearing. Idiopathic sudden hearing loss leads to a decrease in perilymphatic oxygen pressure; using HBO, pressures have been increased by up to 450%.[20]

It works as follows, exposing the patient to 1.5-3 times sea level pressure with 100% oxygen in a specialised hyperbaric chamber, at a pressure range of 1.5-2 atmospheres absolute to 2.4-2.5 in rescue therapy, for approximately one to two hours per session.[21]

It has been proposed for use as an initial therapy within the first fourteen days of symptom onset or rescue therapy as a recent and innovative therapy. So far, no relevant association has been made between severity of hearing loss and response to HBO, nor have differences in the potential for improvement been demonstrated between patients treated during the first week of symptom onset or the second week, however, if use is started beyond two weeks to four weeks, the potential for recovery decreases. [21]

It has been compared as an add-on therapy to regular steroid medication versus steroid therapy alone and found no difference based on recovery outcomes.

HBO was recently accepted as a rescue therapy, with possibilities for use in a window period of up to one month after symptom onset. The indication is in those who have not demonstrated improvement in hearing, specifically, a gain of less than 20 dB. Currently, because of its new and recent use in sudden idiopathic hearing loss, there are no standardised guidelines or protocols in terms of dosage, frequency or timing of initiation after completion of a previous course of initial therapy, such as an initial course of intratympanic or systemic steroids, including HBO or possible combinations thereof.[22]

It has been used with daily sessions at oxygen pressure doses of 2.4 atmospheres absolute for 20 days or the administration of a total of 21 sessions, one per day over a three-week period. Each session has been of similar duration, approximately 120 minutes, in three periods every 20 minutes plus an extra rest period. Another form of use is for 10 to 20 days at doses of 2.0-2.5 atmospheres absolute with 90 minutes duration of each session. The greatest benefit is obtained with a therapy duration of 1200 minutes, which is the current recommended summed therapy time. However, there are no specifications on the levels of pressure administered, it has not been associated with hearing recovery above certain levels, therefore, the ranges should be kept between: 2.0-2.5 ATA.[23]Improvements in hearing have been documented when using HBO, however, the results from definite improvement have little evidence at present.

The maximum benefit is obtained when the hearing loss is severe or profound. The results obtained have shown that their combined use with steroids provides superior effectiveness compared to the use of either of these two therapies alone. As a percentage, a hearing improvement of 84% can be expressed when combining intratympanic steroid therapy and hyperbaric oxygen during the first two weeks.[24]

Adverse effects and risks include pressure changes, such as pulmonary, sinus or oxygen poisoning; claustrophobia or anxiety related to the confinement required to administer the treatment; failure to equalise middle ear pressures following therapy; and residual Eustachian tube dysfunction. It is an expensive treatment, so the physician and patient must come to a joint agreement on the cost-benefit of the therapy.[25]

By way of comparison and summary, intratympanic steroids and HBO administration are two measures that act differently in the inner ear. Intratympanic steroids reach the inner ear by diffusion through the round window and reduce inflammation; whereas HBO generates diffusion through the blood vessels to increase oxygen directly to the area supplying the inner ear structures. Both have the ability to improve cochlear functionality.

The variable of temporality acquires relevance when treating idiopathic sudden hypoacusis, which is why it continues to be part of the otorhinolaryngologist's emergencies and action must be timely. Steroid therapy substantially decreases its effectiveness when used between 4-6 weeks of symptom onset; on the other hand, HBO manages a similar behaviour, in addition to their limited possibilities for improvement when the patients have not been treated with steroid courses during the first two weeks.[26-]


**Follow-up**


As with any other pathology, and as a potential risk for patient disability and impact on quality of life, and because it involves a sensitive organ that may ultimately limit patients' communication and social interaction, audiometric monitoring should be performed during treatment and within the first six months post-treatment.It is imperative to document improvement, recovery or treatment failure compared to initial pre-treatment audiograms. The comprehensive assessment consists of audiometric thresholds within the pure tone average

(PTA) and speech discrimination (WSR) and proceed to recognise hearing loss recovery.Throughout patient surveillance, there have been different meanings for "recovery" of hearing. In the past, it was preferred only to compare hearing with both PTA and WSR against the healthy ear, which would imply socially functional hearing. Today, although there are still several options for the appropriate meaning, a PTA improvement of 10-30 dB or a 10-20% improvement in speech discrimination persists as a common criterion. Furahashi has proposed assessment measures that include PTA at four frequencies: 500, 1000, 2000, 4000 Hz, and classifies it into three possibilities of improvement: full recovery, PTA less than 25 dB or identical to the unaffected contralateral ear; partial recovery, PTA improvement greater than 30 dB; slight recovery, PTA with improvement between 10-30 dB; and no recovery, PTA with improvement less than 10 dB.[29-30]

Residual hearing can be categorised as either "useful" or "not useful". Useful hearing means that the patient can be rehabilitated with amplifiers and maintains a PTA with a recovery of greater than 10 dB or a WSR with a recovery of greater than 10%; whereas "non-useful" hearing limits the patient's access to this type of therapy.

**Rehabilitation**

Hearing in useful ranges may benefit from the use of amplifiers. Prior to individual selection, it is necessary to carry out tests that provide an overview of the impact of idiopathic sudden hearing loss on the patient's quality of life, such as the "Hearing handicap inventory for the Elderly", the "Hearing handicap inventory for Adults" and the "Tinnitus handicap inventory".[31]
The use of contralateral signal routing hearing aids for unilateral or bilateral use, depending on whether or not there is bilateral hearing damage. Monaural devices and even the possibility of cochlear implantation if the hearing loss is severe or profound and if accompanied by tinnitus.
Rehabilitative management goes hand in hand with the results obtained in the tests mentioned in previous paragraphs, the risk benefit and the cost of the therapy to be provided; all with the possibility of providing improvements in hearing, tinnitus and quality of life.

**Forecast**

The prognosis for hearing improvement, whether partial or total, has been linked to factors such as the age of the patient, the form of initial presentation, the degree of documented hearing loss and the underlying obvious or undetermined aetiology as part of the approach to idiopathic sudden hearing loss.

There is little likelihood of recovery within the first two weeks of symptom onset in those patients whose initial picture is accompanied by vestibular symptomatology, with a flat audiometric pattern or morphologically described as a descending curve pattern, at severe or deep levels or poor speech audiometry results.[32-33]

Elderly patients from 60 years of age onwards are considered a special population in the evolution of the condition, due to the high prevalence of associated comorbidities such as: diabetes mellitus, systemic arterial hypertension, hyperlipidaemia and presbycusis; which interfere with the initial treatment protocol with corticosteroids and, therefore, place them at risk of developing presbycusis, accidents and hearing loss. cerebrovascular disease, Meniere's disease in 4-8% and, alterations in blood glycaemia levels and its associated complications.[34]

In addition, both diabetes mellitus and arterial hypertension are entities that alter the microcirculation at the multi-organ level and, therefore, within the inner ear, which explains why they are poor prognostic factors for the complete or significant recovery of hearing thresholds. Other related factors include the recovery of only about 3.6% when the initial picture presents as profound hearing loss.[35]

The type of hearing loss is another factor involved in the evolution of the condition. Formerly, in 1982, low-frequency sensorineural hearing loss with preservation of high frequencies was classified as a subtype of idiopathic sudden hearing loss. Today, it is integrated as part of the pathophysiology of Meniere's disease and has been associated with a better short-term prognosis after timely treatment.[36]

In conclusion, the poor prognostic factors are: age at presentation, over 40-60 years of age; the audiometric pattern with which the hearing loss initially presents, from profound hearing loss to a descending pattern or poor speech audiometry, and added symptoms, mainly the presence of vertigo. Other factors can also be added, such as underlying comorbidities and the administration of timely treatment that does not put the patient at greater risk for possible adverse effects. [7,10,35, 36]

**Scientific Background**

The Unerseas and Hyperbaric Medical Sociey (UHMS) approved the use of hyperbaric oxygen therapy as a treatment for sudden idiopathic hearing loss in October 2011; although it has been used as a treatment option since 1970, previously approved in 1960 as an adjunctive treatment in Germany and France.[19]

To assess the benefit of therapy as a rescue treatment, Furahashi has proposed evaluation measures that include PTA at four frequencies: 500, 1000, 2000, 4000 Hz, and classifies it into three possibilities of improvement: full recovery, PTA less than 25 dB or identical to the unaffected contralateral ear; partial recovery, PTA improvement greater than 30 dB; slight recovery, PTA with improvement between 10-30 dB; and no recovery, PTA with improvement less than 10 dB.[29-30]

Rhee et al in 2018, conducted a randomised clinical trial comparing the use of hyperbaric oxygen therapy and medical therapy with the use of medical therapy; they analysed 16 studies, a total of 2,401 patients with idiopathic sudden sudden hearing loss, the absolute gain was greater in the group given combined therapy (medical therapy and HBO), with a total duration of HBO therapy of at least 1200 minutes.[22]

On the other hand, Capuano et al, in 2015, conducted a retrospective cohort with 300 diseased ears divided into three groups according to the treatment provided: contribution with intravenous corticosteroids only, therapy with hyperbaric oxygen only and a third group with both therapies combined; the results obtained highlight better hearing gains when the therapy was provided the first 2 weeks after the onset of symptoms, and a greater complete recovery 58% and an 84% response to combined therapies.[24]

# IIIPROBLEM STATEMENT

What is the efficacy of hyperbaric oxygen therapy as a rescue treatment in patients diagnosed with idiopathic sudden hearing loss?

# IV  JUSTIFICATION

The US incidence of idiopathic sudden hearing loss is 5-20 per 100,000 population and a total of 66,000 cases annually. The exact figure in the Mexican population remains unknown. For this reason, the present study will focus on the investigation of this pathology in Mexico.

This work will show the efficacy of hyperbaric oxygen therapy as a rescue treatment for the return of hearing, since this disease causes serious morbidity in the patient who suffers from it; it leads to disability of the individual in their daily life activities and compromises their quality of life by preventing adequate social interaction and communication, a problem that extends both in the short and long term. The aim is to improve the prognosis for hearing recovery and avoid any possibility of chronic damage and long-term disability.

Correct identification of such an emergency and timely treatment within the first few days of symptom onset is imperative, however, when more than two weeks have passed, the chances of hearing recovery diminish and therapeutic options are limited. An innovative option for rescue treatment is hyperbaric oxygen therapy, which has shown benefits in absolute hearing restoration of 5 to 12 dB[23] , however, the dosage and frequency is still in the process of standardisation. For this reason, the present research focuses on comparative hearing before and after treatment, and will contribute to the evidence of the efficacy of this therapy.

To carry out the study, the otorhinolaryngology and head and neck surgery service of the Civil Hospital of Culiacán has the facilities to provide hyperbaric oxygen therapy, hearing studies and records of patients previously treated with hyperbaric oxygen.The study formally complies with the research policies of the Centro de Investigación y Docencia en Ciencias de la Salud and the Hospital Civil de Culiacán and has therefore been approved.

# V  HYPOTHESIS

Patients with idiopathic sudden sudden hearing loss who undergo rescue treatment with hyperbaric oxygen therapy will achieve a full or moderate degree of recovery.

# VI  OBJECTIVES

## 7.1. Objective general

To establish the efficacy of hyperbaric oxygen therapy in confirmed patients with idiopathic sudden sudden hearing loss.

## 7.2. Objectives specific.

**7.2.1.** To identify the degree of hearing recovery in patients with idiopathic sudden hearing loss.

**7.2.2.** To assess the presence of hearing improvement in patients with idiopathic sudden sudden hearing loss.

**7.2.3.** To assess the degree of hearing loss in patients with idiopathic sudden hearing loss.

**7.2.4.** Identify the laterality of the affected ear.

**7.2.5.** To quantify the time of evolution of idiopathic sudden sudden hearing loss.

**7.2.6.** To assess the presence of adverse effects of hyperbaric oxygen therapy.

**VII MATERIALS AND METHODS**

**8.1. Design of the study**

**Taxonomy:** observational, descriptive, retrospective.
**Type of study:** Cohort.

**8.2. Universe of the study:** the clinical records of patients who attended for consultation at the otorhinolaryngology and Head and Neck Surgery service diagnosed with idiopathic sudden hypoacusis.

**8.3. Venue:** Hospital Civil de Culiacán.

**8.4. Implementation period:** March 2020 to July 2023.

**8.5. Criteria for inclusion:**

Age 18 years or older.
Both sexes.
With a diagnosis of confirmed idiopathic sudden hearing loss.
With an evolution of the clinical picture of at least two weeks, in spite of having received initial treatment or none at all.

**8.6. exclusion criteria**

Patients with a diagnosis of sensorineural hearing loss with an identifiable cause.
Patients with clinical signs of neurological involvement.
Patients with concomitant disease such as: Eustachian tube dysfunction, traumatic brain injury, Meniere's disease, labyrinthitis, migraine, vestibular neuronitis, serous otitis media.

22

Patients with previous ear surgery.

Inability to perform hyperbaric oxygen therapy.

## 8.7. Criteria for elimination

Dropout from hyperbaric oxygen therapy, who have not completed 10 sessions.

Lack of audiometric monitoring, for whatever reason, before and after completing 10 sessions of hyperbaric oxygen.

Concomitant eventuality during therapies: vertiginous syndrome, serous otitis media or tympanic perforation.

## 8.8. Analysis statistical:

For continuous variables, descriptive statistical measures were used: central tendency and data dispersion. In the case of categorical variables, percentages and frequencies will be used. Continuous variables will be compared with Student's t-test and categorical variables with chi-square. P:S0.05 will be considered statistically significant.

**8.9. Sample size calculation:** N=93 for 95% confidence interval. Formula for a proportion.

A convenience sample was taken. All patient records meeting the inclusion criteria, in the period from March 2020 to July 2023, will be included.

**8.10. General description of the study Patient recruitment.**

Patients attending the Otorhinolaryngology and Head and Neck Surgery Service of the Civil Hospital of Culiacán who were diagnosed with sudden sensorineural hearing loss by interrogation, physical examination and complete hearing study were included. During March 2020 to July 2023.

**Data collection.**

A data collection sheet was drawn up according to the variables obtained in the review. of clinical records.

**Timing and frequency of measurements.**

The main instrument to objectively verify the variables retrospectively in patients with idiopathic sudden hypoacusis was audiometry before and after the 10 hyperbaric oxygen therapies, data that we will collect from the clinical file.

**Data reporting.**

Once the data has been collected, it will be exported from the Excel spreadsheet to the SPSS statistical package for organisation, coding and the proposed statistical analysis. Once the statistical analysis of the data has been completed, the results will be critically interpreted and then the discussion and conclusions of the study will be drawn.

**Flow chart.**

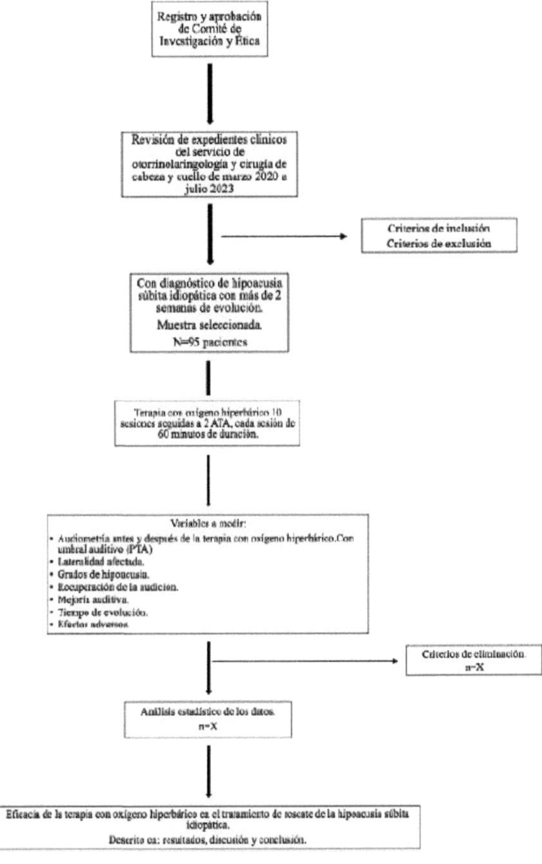



Figure 1. Flow chart.

**8.11. Table of operational definition of variables Independent variable:** hyperbaric oxygen therapy. **Dependent variable:** degree of hearing recovery.

Table 1. Summary of variables.

| Variable | Definition Operational | Variable Type | Scale Of Measurement |
|---|---|---|---|
| | This is when the patient with idiopathic sudden hearing loss has a hearing restoration after hyperbaric oxygen therapy. | | |
| Of interest primary: | It is measured: | | |
| Degree of hearing recovery | Complete: return of hearing within 15 dB of the unaffected or contralateral ear. | Qualitative | Ordinal |
| | Moderate: improvement of more than 10 dB, but not back within 15 dB of the unaffected ear. | | |
| | Poor: Hearing level unchanged, improvement less than or equal to 10dB or deterioration after treatment. Success: when the patient shows a complete or moderate recovery. Failure: when the patient presents a poor recovery. | | |
| Of interest secondary: Hearing improvement | No/Yes. | Qualitative | Nominal |

| | | | |
|---|---|---|---|
| Degree of hearing loss | It is measured with a scale, according to the pure tone average obtained by audiometry (PTA) averaged over the frequencies 500, 1000 and 2000 Hz: Surface: 20-40 dB | Qualitative | Ordinal |
| | Moderate: 41 to 60 dBSevere: 61-80 dB Deep: 81-100 dB | | |
| Laterality of the affected ear | Left/Right. | Qualitative | Nominal |
| Time course of sudden hearing loss idiopathic | It is measured in months and days. | Quantitative | Continua |
| Adverse effects of hyperbaric oxygen therapy | It is when the patient with idiopathic sudden hypoacusis treated with hyperbaric oxygen as rescue treatment presents an undesirable effect: middle ear barotrauma, para nasal sinus barotrauma. Management: Withdrawal from therapy, follow up in outpatient clinic. | Qualitative | Nominal. |
| Idiopathic sudden hearing loss. | This is when the patient presents with a rapid and unexplained hearing loss of sensorineural aetiology occurring within a 72-hour window period, a decrease in hearing of more than 30 dB affecting at least 3 consecutive frequencies. | Qualitative | Nominal |

**8.12. Standardisation of measuring instruments**

Audiometer: Interacustic, Ad629 Audiometer and Mt10 tympanometer.

Scale for measuring degree of hearing loss: According to the classification in decibels (dB) of the Mexican Clinical Practice Guideline "Hipoacusia Súbita Sensorineural Idiopática". 2010.

Scale for measuring hearing improvement: As proposed in the article: Hyperbaric oxygen therapy in treatment of sudden sensorineural hearing loss: finding for the maximal therapeutic benefit of different applied pressures. UHM 2019.

Scale for measuring the degree of hearing recovery: As proposed in the Clinical practice guideline: sudden hearing loss. Otolaryngol-Head Neck Surg Off J Am Acad Otolaryngol-Head Neck Surg 2012, citing the article "Efficacy of hyperbaric oxygen therapy as a supplementary therapy of sudden sensorineural hearing loss in the Slovak Republic" by Krajcovicova et al 2018.

**8.13. Registration of protocol with the Research Committee and Research Ethics Committee.**

The present work entitled "Efficacy of hyperbaric oxygen therapy in the rescue treatment of idiopathic sudden hypoacusis" was evaluated and approved by the RESEARCH COMMITTEE (REGISTRATION: 19 CI 25 006 004) with Dr. Saúl Armando Beltrán Ontiveros as chairman of the committee; on 14 May 2023 with approval number 451.

The present work entitled "Efficacy of hyperbaric oxygen therapy in the rescue treatment of sudden idiopathic hypoacusis" was evaluated and approved by the RESEARCH ETHICS COMMITTEE (Registration before the National Bioethics Commission: CONBIOETHICS-25-CEI-001-20180523) with Dr. Martha Elvia Quiñonez Meza as president of the committee; on 03 July 2023 with approval number 129-2023.

**Human resources:** For the development of this research project, resident doctors from the Otorhinolaryngology and Head and Neck Surgery Service of the Civil Hospital of Culiacán, doctors assigned to the service, interns in social service and support from the nursing staff of the service and social work were involved.

**Physical resources:** outpatient facilities of the Otorhinolaryngology and Head and Neck Surgery service. Clinical archive of the Civil Hospital of Culiacán, to include medical treatments and pre- and post-hyperbaric chamber hearing studies.

**Material resources:** SPSS system, data collection sheet of recruited patients.to the study, informed consents.

**Funding:** not required for this research study as it is retrospective.

A total of 38 files were collected where data related to neurotological pathology were obtained; the main requirement was to have suffered from idiopathic sudden hypoacusis and to have been confirmed by hearing studies with no other underlying cause, and the second requirement was to have received treatment with hyperbaric oxygen therapy as a rescue treatment for hearing improvement.The age range of the affected ear was between 26 and 75 years of age, with a mean of 51.4±12.2 years; the incidence was predominantly in females with 60.5% (23), compared to males, 39.5% (15). The frequency of involvement between both ears was similar, with the left ear being affected 55.3% (21) and the right ear 44.7% (17).Before the start of hyperbaric oxygen therapy, the medical history of each patient was assessed in detail. 39.4% (15) had no relevant medical history; however, the remaining 60.5% (23) had other medical history to consider in neurootological pathology, such as: hypertension 15.7% (6), diabetes mellitus type 2 with 15.7% (6), obesity 2.6% (1), smoking 5.2% (2), alcoholism 5.2% (2), benign paroxysmal positional vertigo 5.2% (2),contralateral congenital hearing loss 2.6% (1), contralateral acoustic trauma 2.6% (1), contralateral acoustic syndrome2.6% (1) and depression 2.6% (1).Likewise, 42.8% (6 out of 14) of the patients with comorbidities presented one or more of these factors; some frequent associations: smoking with hypertension or type 2 diabetes mellitus, type 2 diabetes mellitus with hypertension, hypertension and alcoholism, or a surplus of depression and contralateral acoustic trauma. While the remaining 57.1% (8 out of 14) had only one co-morbidity. The above was considered for the description of the findings in order to correlate possible underlying risk factors.

Table 2. General characteristics.

| Features | Population of study |
|---|---|
| No. of patients | 38 |
| Age, mean±SD (years) | 51.4±12.2 |
| Female sex (%) | 60.5 |
| Male sex (%) | 39.5 |
| Right ear (%) | 44.7 |
| Left ear (%) | 55.3 |
| HBO pre-treatment (%) | |
| Intratympanic corticosteroid (%) | 97.4 |
| Dexamethasone | 86.8 |
| Methylprednisolone | 7.9 |
| Dexametsone+methylprednisolone | 2.6 |
| Systemic corticosteroid (%) | 73.7 |
| Prednisone | 68.4 |
| Deflazacort | 5.2 |
| Comorbidities (%) | |
| Diabetes mellitus type 2 | 15.7 |
| Arterial Hypertension | 15.7 |
| Obesity | 2.6 |
| Depression | 2.6 |
| Smoking | 5.2 |
| Alcoholism | 5.2% |
| ENT history (%) | |
| Ramsay Hunt Syndrome | 2.6 |
| Acoustic trauma (contralateral) | 2.6 |
| Congenital hearing loss (contralateral) | 2.6 |
| Benign paroxysmal positional vertigo | 5.2 |

SD: standard deviation, HBO: hyperbaric oxygen.

Despite the treatment provided as hyperbaric oxygen rescue, data were analysed in relation to the previous treatment provided and described in the literature, both the use of systemic and intratympanic corticosteroids, together with the rescue treatment. In this study, 23.7% (9) received treatment with intratympanic corticosteroids; 73.7% (28) received treatment with both oral corticosteroids at the systemic and intratympanic level, and one third received rescue treatment with oral corticosteroids at the intratympanic level, and one third received rescue treatment with oral corticosteroids at the intratympanic level. 2.6% (1) with no previous treatment, who were attempted to receive rescue treatment with hyperbaric oxygen only, given the time of evolution. None of the files analysed received systemic steroid alone

31

prior to rescue therapy.It was also found that the most commonly used systemic corticosteroid was prednisone in 68.4% (26), followed by deflazacort in 5.2% (2) (Table 2.).) The most commonly used corticosteroid in intratympanic treatment w a s  dexamethasone in 86.8% (33), followed b y  methylprednisolone in 7.9% (3), 1 patient (2.6%) received combined infiltrations with dexamethasone and methylprednisolone.Subsequently, the analysis of the hyperbaric oxygen therapy itself was collected, where files had previously been selected that complied with at least 10 sessions of hyperbaric oxygen therapy, each lasting a minimum of 60 minutes, and under the stipulations for the use of this therapy as a rescue treatment for idiopathic sudden hypoacusis, i.e. at least 2 weeks had passed since the onset of symptoms, without improvement after intratympanic or systemic treatment with corticosteroids; or without previous treatment. Under these statutes, an improvement of more than 10 dB was obtained in 63.2% (24); complete recovery in 26.3% (10), moderate recovery in 36.8% (14) and poor recovery in 36.8% (14). (Figure 2,table 3-5)

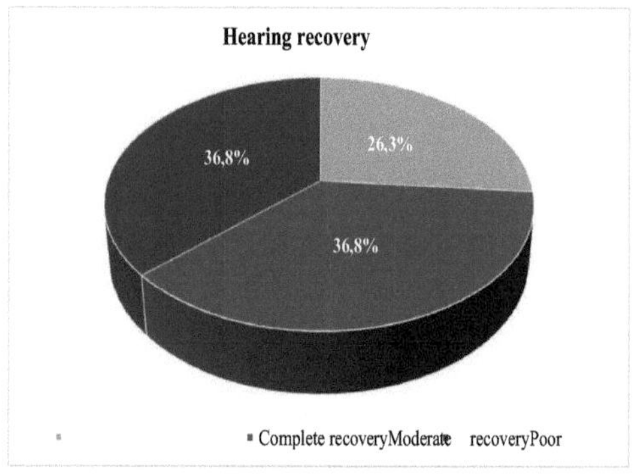


Figure 2. Hearing recovery graph.

Table 3. Decibel matched samples.

|  | Mean±DE pre HBO (dB) | Mean±DE post HBO (dB) | Difference (dB) | Sig. |
|---|---|---|---|---|
| PTA | 63.4±23.7 | 48.1±27.5 | 15.3 | .000 |

SD: standard deviation, dB: decibels, Sig: significance, PTA: pure tone average.

Table 4. Hearing improvement

| Hearing improvement | Percentage (n) |
| --- | --- |
| With hearing improvement | 63.2% (24) |
| No hearing improvement | 36.8% (14) |
| TOTAL | 100% (38) |

n: number of patients.

Table 5. Hearing recovery.

| Degrees of hearing recovery | Percentage (n) |
| --- | --- |
| Full recovery | 26.3% (10) |
| Moderate recovery | 36.8% (14) |
| Poor recovery | 36.8% (14) |
| TOTAL | 100% (38) |

n: number of patients.

The average of pure tones before and after therapy was an indicator for this analysis and an overall gain of 15.3 dB (p .000) was evident, concluding a mean in dB pre hyperbaric chamber of 63.4 ± 23.7 dB and post hyperbaric chamber of 48.1 ± 27.5 dB.The time from the onset of the clinical picture to the start of hyperbaric oxygen therapy was correlated with the decibel gain in hearing described in the previous paragraphs, described in weeks; the results were an overall mean of 8.8+/-19.8 weeks. In the 26.3% with complete hearing recovery the mean in weeks was 4 ± 4; in the moderate recovery (36.8%), 7.1 ± 9.8 weeks, and in the poor recovery section, 14 ± 31 weeks.There was a trend in greater hearing gain in decibels when providing therapy over an average of at least 4 weeks, as a calculated average. As shown in table 6 and figure 4.

Table 6. Hearing recovery at the time of initiation of hyperbaric oxygen therapy.

| Degrees of recovery | % (n) | Mean±DE (weeks) Initiation of hyperbaric oxygen therapy |
| --- | --- | --- |
| Full recovery | 26.3 (10) | 4 ± 4 |
| Moderate recovery | 36.8 (14) | 7.1 ± 9.8 |
| Poor recovery | 36.8 (14) | 4 ± 31 |

n: number of patients, SD: standard deviation.

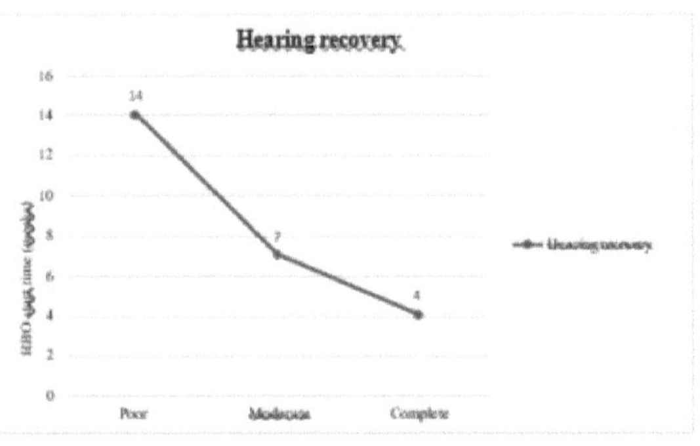


Figure 3. Hearing recovery at the time of initiation of hyperbaric oxygen therapy.

HBO: Hyperbaric oxygen.

Those who started hyperbaric oxygen therapy with a profound hearing loss (>80 dB), 22.2% improved to a lesser degree of hearing loss between 60-80 dB, 2.22% improved to a mild degree of hearing loss, leaving 55.6% within the same classification. Those who were classified as having severe hearing loss (60-80 dB) prior to therapy improved 41.7% to moderate hearing loss, 16.7% to mild hearing loss, 16.7% to normal hearing loss (<20 dB) and 25% remained unchanged. Moderate hearing loss (40-60 dB) had 11 patients of the records collected, of which 45.5% improved to a mild degree of hearing loss and 9.1% recovered normal hearing; the remaining 4 patients (36.4%) in the category remained with moderate hearing loss. And of the last 4 who were reported to have mild hearing loss (20-40 dB) before starting therapy, 75% achieved normal hearing at the end of therapy, while 25% remained with a mild degree of hearing loss.Overall the percentage of patients with profound hearing loss pre hyperbaric chamber decreased from 23.6% to 13.2%, severe hearing loss improved from 31.5% pre chamber to 15.8% post, moderate hearing loss pre therapy totaled 28.9%, which decreased to a total of 23.7%. While those with mild hearing loss had a change from 10.5% to 10% post hyperbaric chamber. (Table 7.)

Table 7. Cross-tabulation of degrees of hypoaucusia pre and post hyperbaric chamber.

| | Post-HBO <20dB | Post-HBO 20-40dB | Post-HBO 40-60 dB | Post-HBO 60-80 dB | Post-HBO >80 dB | TOTAL Pre-HBO |
|---|---|---|---|---|---|---|
| Pre-HBO <20dB | 100% (2) | 0% | 0% | 0% | 0% | 5.2 % (2) |
| Pre-HBO 20-40dB | 75% (3) | 25% (1) | 0% | 0% | 0% | 10.5% (4) |
| Pre-HBO 40-60 dB | 9.1% (1) | 45.5% (5) | 36.4% (4) | 9.1% (1) | 0% | 28.9% (11) |
| Pre-HBO 60-80 dB | 16.7% (2) | 16.7% (2) | 41.7% (5) | 25% (3) | 0% | 31.5% (12) |
| Pre-HBO >80 dB | 0% | 22.2% (2) | 0% | 22.2% (2) | 55.6% (5) | 23.6% (9) |
| TOTAL Post-HBO | 21.1% (8) | 26.3% (10) | 23.7% (9) | 15.8% (6) | 13.2% (5) | 38 |

dB: decibels, HBO: hyperbaric oxygen.

The distribution in auditory frequencies to analyse in depth the auditory gains, showed a higher recovery in 500 Hz, being 17.1±21.5 dB, followed by 250 Hz with a recovery of 14.7±21.4 dB and in third place in gain were 1000Hz and 6000 Hz with 14.2±18.1 dB and 14.2±19.9 dB, respectively. The most affected frequencies prior to hyperbaric oxygen therapy were predominantly high frequencies: 4000, 6000 and 8000 Hz with means of 69±28.1 dB, 69.4±28.5dB and 72.7±29.8 dB, respectively. The least affected frequencies prior to the start of therapy were 125 Hz with 46.03±22.2 dB; 250 Hz with 52.8±25.2 dB and 500 Hz with 60±27.1 dB. Within the same data it was observed that 4 patients at the frequency of 125 Hz were not able to detect any stimulus, similar with the frequency of 250 Hz, where one of them showed no response (Table 8.) (Figure 3.).

Table 8. Frequency hearing gain (dB).

| Frequency (Hz) | Mean±DE pre HBO (dB) | Mean±DE post HBO (dB) | Hearing improvement (mean±De) (dB) | 95% CI | Sig. |
|---|---|---|---|---|---|
| 125 | 46.03±22.2 | 34.5±22.5 | 11.4±18.6 | 4.9-17.9 | .001 |
| 250 | 52.8±25.2 | 27.7±20.4 | 25.1±21.8 | 17.8-32.4 | .000 |
| 500 | 60±27.1 | 42.8±27.6 | 17.1±21.5 | 10-24.1 | .000 |
| 1000 | 62.7±26.5 | 48.5±29.5 | 14.2±18.1 | 8.2-20.1 | .000 |
| 2000 | 65.5±26.6 | 52.5±30.4 | 13±18.4 | 6.9-19 | .000 |
| 3000 | 66±26.6 | 53.8±29.3 | 12.2±17.6 | 6.4-18 | .000 |
| 4000 | 69±28.1 | 57.1±30.5 | 11.9±14.3 | 7.2-16.6 | .000 |
| 6000 | 69.4±28.5 | 55.2±30.8 | 14.2±19.9 | 7.6-20.7 | .000 |
| 8000 | 72.7±29.8 | 62.6±30.7 | 10±16.8 | 4.6-15.6 | .001 |

Hz: hertz, SD: standard deviation, dB: decibels, CI: confidence interval, Sig: Significance.

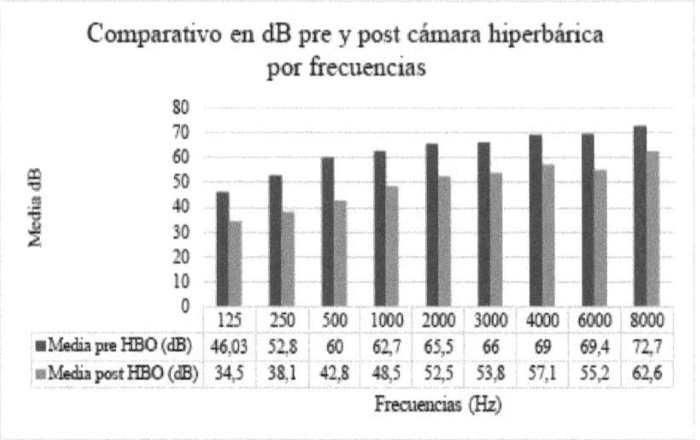


| | 125 | 250 | 500 | 1000 | 2000 | 3000 | 4000 | 6000 | 8000 |
|---|---|---|---|---|---|---|---|---|---|
| Media pre HBO (dB) | 46,03 | 52,8 | 60 | 62,7 | 65,5 | 66 | 69 | 69,4 | 72,7 |
| Media post HBO (dB) | 34,5 | 38,1 | 42,8 | 48,5 | 52,5 | 53,8 | 57,1 | 55,2 | 62,6 |

Figure 4. Hearing gain at different frequencies.

Hz: hertz, dB: decibels, HBO: hyperbaric oxygen.

In itself an improvement and recovery of hearing as catalogued on audiometry were the predominant main criteria to be assessed, however, additional descriptive data on hearing gain after therapy was collected when comparing speech audiometry studies; 57.8%(22) obtained an improvement in the percentage and decibels perceived by the affected ear, and 42.1% (22) obtained an improvement in the percentage and decibels perceived by the affected ear.(16) unchanged from the study prior to hyperbaric oxygen therapy (Table 9).

Table 9. Improvement in speech audiometry and speech perception.

| Speech audiometry | Percentage (n) |
|---|---|
| Improvement in speech audiometry | 57.8 (22) |
| No change in speech audiometry | 42.1 (16) |
| TOTAL | 100% (38) |

n: number of patients.

In addition to the above, a more extensive analysis of changes in speech audiometry was performed. As can be seen in Table 10 below, of the 22 patients (57.8%) who showed changes towards improvement in speech audiometric uptake, 18 of them had 100% uptake at a range from 25 to 80 dB, which is a noteworthy feature in cases of spoken language perception, communication and improvements in the quality of life of the patients.

Table 10. Improvements in speech audiometry.

| PATIENT | PRE HBO SPEECH AUDIOMETRY | POST HBO SPEECH AUDIOMETRY |
|---|---|---|
| 1. | 0% to 100 dB | 75% to 90 dB |
| 2. | 40% at 90 dB | 100% at 40 dB |
| 3. | 0% to 100 dB | 100% at 80 dB |
| 4. | 100% at 90 dB | 100% at 70 dB |
| 5. | 100% at 45 dB | 100% at 25 dB |
| 6. | 0% to 100 dB | 100% at 45 dB |
| 7. | 0% at 70 dB | 100% at 80 dB |
| 8. | 0% to 100 dB | 100% at 50 dB |
| 9. | 100% at 75 dB | 100% at 60 dB |
| 10. | 80% at 50 dB | 100% at 45 dB |
| 11. | 100% at 70 dB | 100% at 50 dB |
| 12. | 100% at 80 dB | 100% at 60 dB |
| 13. | 40% at 75 dB | 80% at 60 dB |
| 14. | 100% at 35 dB | 100% at 30 dB |
| 15. | 20% at 100 dB | 60% at 90 dB |
| 16. | 90% at 70 dB | 100% at 40 dB |
| 17. | 0% to 100 dB | 100% at 50 dB |
| 18. | 100% at 60 dB | 100% at 30 dB |
| 19. | 60% at 90 dB | 100% at 80 dB |
| 20. | 100% at 100 dB | 100% at 50 dB |
| 21. | 40% at 105 dB | 70% at 100 dB |
| 22. | No catchment | 100% at 60 dB |

HBO: hyperbaric oxygen, dB: decibels.

After analysis of the hearing gains themselves, they were related to the treatment they had previously received and it was found that of the 24 who had hearing improvement, 25% (6 out of 24) were treated with intratympanic corticosteroids, and 75% (18 out of 24) were previously treated with a simultaneous combination of intratympanic and systemic corticosteroids. It was noted that the patient who had no pre-treatment prior to rescue therapy had no hearing improvement, 7.1% (1 of 14); the remaining 21.4% (3 of 14) and 71.4% (10 of 14) had received intratympanic corticosteroid injections and both systemic and intratympanic therapies, respectively.Likewise those with complete hearing recovery (10), 30% (3 out of 10) received previous intratympanic therapy, and 70% (7 out of 10) combined intratympanic and systemic therapy. With moderate recovery (14), the majority 78.5% (11 out of 14) were given combined therapy and 21.4% (3 out of 14) had only received previous intratympanic therapy.

Finally, those with poor recovery, 71.4% (10 of 14) received combined therapy, 21.4% (3 of 14) prior intratympanic therapy, and 7.1% (1 of 14) did not receive therapy prior to salvage treatment. (Table 11-13.) (Figure 5-7.)

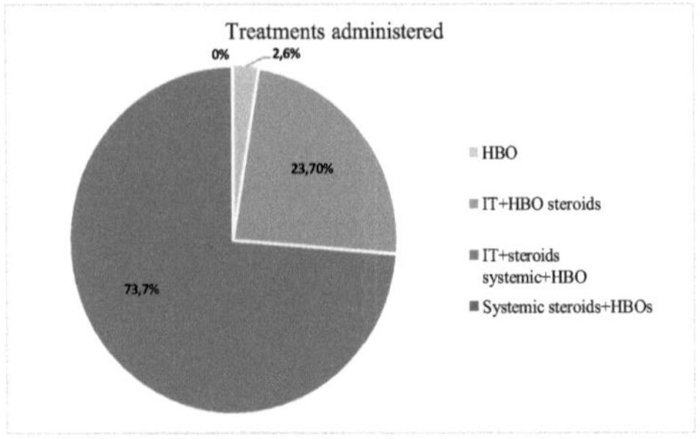


Figure 5. Treatments administered.

HBO: hyperbaric oxygen, IT: intra-tympanic.

Table 11. Treatments administered.

| Treatments administered | Percentage (n) |
| --- | --- |
| HBO | 2.6 (1) |
| IT+HBO steroids | 23.7 (9) |
| IT+steroids systemic+HBO | 73.7 (28) |
| Systemic steroids+HBOs | 0 (0) |
| TOTAL | 100% (38) |

n: number of patients, HBO: hyperbaric oxygen, IT: intrathympanic.

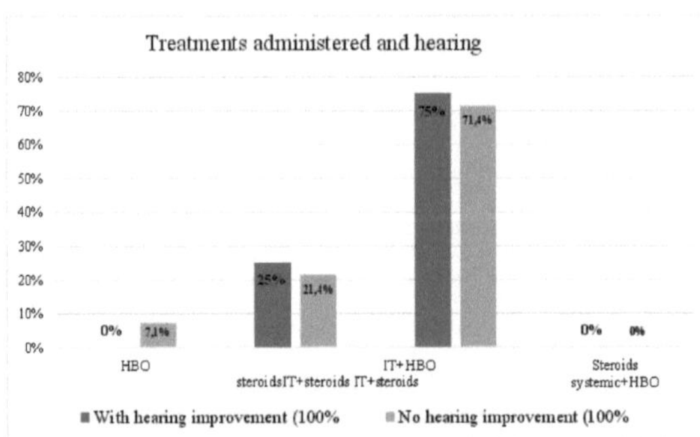


Figure 6. Treatments administered and hearing improvement.

n: number of patients, HBO: hyperbaric oxygen, IT: intrathympanic.

Table 12. Treatments administered and hearing improvement.

| Treatments administered | With hearing improvement % (n) | No hearing improvement % (n) |
| --- | --- | --- |
| HBO | 0 (0) | 7.1 (1) |
| IT+HBO steroids | 25 (6) | 21.4 (3) |
| IT+steroids systemic+HBO | 75 (18) | 71.4 (10) |
| Systemic steroids+HBOs | 0 (0) | 0 (0) |
| TOTAL | 100% (24) | 100% (14) |

n: number of patients, HBO: hyperbaric oxygen, IT: intrathympanic.

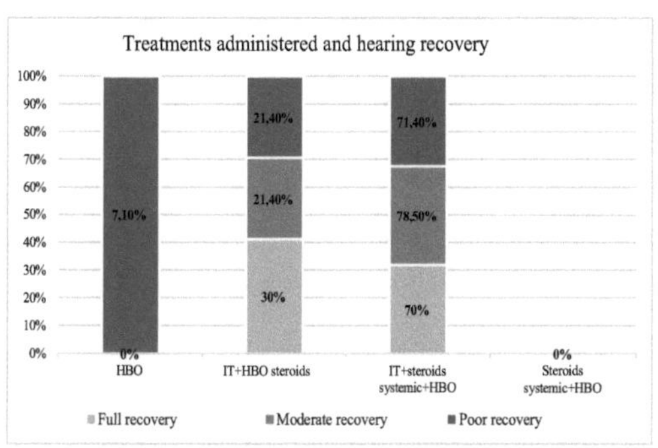


Figure 7. Treatments administered and hearing recovery.

HBO: hyperbaric oxygen, IT: intra-tympanic.

Table 13. Treatments administered and hearing recovery.

| Treatments administered | Full recovery % (n) | Moderate recovery % (n) | Poor recovery % (n) |
| --- | --- | --- | --- |
| HBO | 0 (0) | 0 (0) | 7.1 (1) |
| IT+HBO steroids | 30 (3) | 21.4 (3) | 21.4 (3) |
| IT+steroids systemic+HBO | 70 (7) | 78.5 (11) | 71.4 (10) |
| Steroids systemic+HBO | 0 (0) | 0 (0) | 0 (0) |
| TOTAL | 100 (10) | 100 (14) | 100 (14) |

n: number of patients, HBO: hyperbaric oxygen, IT: intrathympanic.

Among other characteristics collected for the research, complications following hyperbaric oxygen therapy were taken into consideration, where 76.3%, i.e. 29 patients without complications, were recorded. The complications observed were: vertigo in 7.9% of patients. (3); residual tinnitus in 13.1% (5), and tympanic perforation in 2.6% (1). (Figure 8, Table14.)

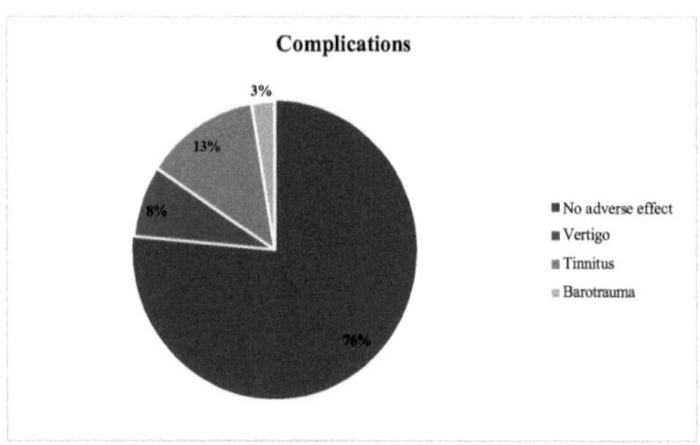


Figure 8. Complications following HBO.

Table 14. Complications following HBO.

| Complication | Percentage (n) |
| --- | --- |
| No adverse effect | 76.3% (29) |
| Vertigo | 7.8% (3) |
| Tinnitus | 13.1% (5) |
| Barotrauma | 2.6% (1) |
| TOTAL | 38 |

n: number of patients.

# X   DISCUSSION

This study focused on the efficacy of hyperbaric oxygen therapy in idiopathic sudden sudden hearing loss, investigating factors such as: degree of hearing loss, laterality of the disease, time of initiation of hyperbaric oxygen therapy, degree of hearing recovery, hearing improvement and the various adverse effects encountered.

Within the data obtained there were a total of 38 files collected and analysed retrospectively, different demographic data to highlight were found, the first of them with respect to sex, where the female sex predominated with 60.5% compared to the male sex where the pathology was less frequent with the remaining percentage of 39.5%; however this difference has not been reported by the literature, it is expected that this has an equal distribution between both sexes. [4,16, 24.]

The peak incidence was between 26 and 75 years, with a mean of 51.4±12.2 years, similar to other studies addressing this pathology. [4,35,23.] The most affected ear was the left ear at 55.3%, however there was no notable difference with the right ear, a fact already commented in the results of Cho et al and Wen et al, the laterality of the disease remains similar between both ears with the exception of 5% with possible bilateral affection, a characteristic that was not possible to see in this study. [35,36.]

Multiple therapies for this condition have been described, however the possible improvement with hyperbaric oxygen is still a matter of debate, there is currently no consensus on the number of sessions required for hearing improvement, the time required for improvement or the degree of pressure in ATA to allow an increase in oxygen pressure within the microvasculature of the inner ear, however the range is between 10-20 sessions of 30-100 minutes each; however the range is between 10-20 sessions lasting between 30 to 100 minutes each, and even more than 20 sessions have been documented and an exposure of between 2.0 to 2.5 ATA. (Table 15). And as a safety limit exposure up to a maximum of 3 ATA. [19,23,37-39.]

Table 15. Previous studies with HBO.

| AUTOR | | | | RESULTADOS | | | |
|---|---|---|---|---|---|---|---|
| | PERIODO DEL ESTUDIO | NO. PACIENTES | CARACTERISTICAS DEL ESTUDIO | Recuperación completa | Recuperación moderada | Pobre recuperación | Media de ganancia (dB) |
| Ohno et al. (2010) | 2001-2008 | 48 | 2.0 ATA por 10 sesiones 60 min cada una. | 2% (1/48) | 28.8% (10/48) | 77% (37/48) | 5.2 |
| Liu et al (2011) | 1999-2009 | 112 | 2.5 ATA por 10-20 sesiones de 60 min cada una | 15.2% (17/12) | 50% (56/112) | 34.8% (39/112) | 24.5 |
| Alimoglu et al. (2011) | 2004-2010 | 61 | 2.5 ATA por 20 sesiones 120 min cada una | 42.6% (26/61) | 22.9% (14/61) | 34.4% (21/61) | 36.8 |
| Yang et al. (2013) | 2013 | 19 | 2 ATA por 20 sesiones de 60 min cada una | 68.4% (13/19) | -- | 31.6% (1-19) | 18.7 |
| Pezzoli et al. (2015) | 2011-2013 | 23 | 2.5 ATA por 15 sesiones 30 min cada una. | 4.3% (1/23) | 21.7% (5/23) | 73.9% (17/23) | 15.6 |
| Psillas (2015) | 2013-2015 | 15 | 2.2 ATA por 15 sesiones a 90 min cada una | 6.6% (1/15) | 40% (6/15) | 53.3% (8/15) | 12.1 |
| Hosokawa et al. (2017) | 2011-2015 | 167 | 1.5 ATA por 10 sesiones de 60 min cada una. | 9.6% (16/167) | 26.9% (45/167) | 63.4% (106/167) | >10 |

ATA: absolute atmospheres, HBO: hyperbaric oxygen, min: minutes, dB: decibels.

Historically, hyperbaric oxygen therapy began to be used in 1960, and during

in 2011 was approved by The Underseas and Hyperbaric Medical Society for use as a treatment for idiopathic sudden hypoacusis.[19] And it has been accepted as rescue or salvage therapy when at least one month has passed since the onset of symptoms, more specifically its use within the first 2 weeks of clinical evolution, as a primary treatment. [22]

The overall decibel gain was 15.3 dB (p= .000), and as documented by the American Academy of Otolaryngology-Head and Neck Surgery Sudden Idiopathic Hearing Loss Guidelines, two measures were taken as a baseline classification of the total data obtained.[11] The first to be described was "hearing improvement" considered as a recovery of at least 10 dB or more, in this study 63.2% had improvement, with the remaining 36.8% with improvement of less than 10 dB. [11,40-43].

As a second descriptive section, the classification of "hearing recovery" was taken in three levels: complete, moderate or poor recovery, as the guide classification reported by Capuano et al. Complete recovery accounted for 26.3% of the total analysed, moderate, 36.8% and poor 36.8%. As discussed in studies by Capuano et al, full recovery has been seen to predominate when hyperbaric oxygen is added to the treatment, i.e. by providing combined treatment, 58% complete recovery is then expressed, compared to only hyperbaric oxygen, 24%, and the use of systemic corticosteroid therapy, 20%. [11,24, 40-43]

As has also been stipulated by other authors such as Pezzoli et al, Psillas et al, Capuano et al or Liu et al; whose studies also took a treatment regimen of at least 10 sessions of hyperbaric oxygen therapy, show our results in 26.3% (patients with complete recovery of hearing, as well as comparing the number of sessions, minutes of each session and pressure in absolute atmospheres (ATA) to which the patients are exposed, data that still remain without stipulated consensus, and scope that merits further research in this regard.

It is also comparable to the hearing gains described by other authors as shown in table 15. This shows multiple investigations that have collected results regarding the use of hyperbaric oxygen therapy as a rescue treatment in idiopathic sudden hearing loss. It shows how the study by Ohno et al found a recovery of approximately 5 dB, with full recovery of only 2%; very variable data to consider other authors, whose hyperbaric chamber protocol was similar, but the gains were up to 24 dB [40,41.] , with full recovery in 15.2%, or Alimoglu et al with maximum gains of up to 36 dB, and full recovery in 42.6% of their patients.

However, when collecting these data and analysing them, our present study obtained a gain very similar to that found and reported by Pezzoli et al, where the gain in decibels was 15 dB; as shown by our data already described in previous paragraphs, where we have obtained a mean in dB pre hyperbaric chamber of $63.4 \pm 23.7$ dB and post hyperbaric chamber of $48.1 \pm 27.5$ dB and a gain in decibels of 15.3 dB. Likewise, our results can be evaluated with respect to the recovery percentages, where the literature describes variable complete recovery, maximum up to 68.4% of the patients and minimum of 2%; however, in the present study we obtained 26.3%; close to the percentage obtained by Liu et al, with 15.2% (Table 15).

Continuing with the analysis, moderate recovery has been reported in up to 50% of patients undergoing hyperbaric oxygen therapy (Table 15.) and poor recovery with high percentages of up to 77%. Our results described moderate and poor recovery with the same percentages, 26.3%, very close to that described by Pezzoli et al, with 21.7% for moderate recovery, and Yang et al, with 31.6%. However, these data are variable with respect to the lack of consensus on the dosage, timing and analysis of hearing recovery for patients undergoing rescue therapy with hyperbaric oxygen.Currently, there is no consensus on the timing of the use of different therapies; it is not yet known exactly how long the maximum interval after the onset of symptoms is when treatment is effective, taking into account the duration of the inflammatory process or vasoconstriction in the inner ear. Several systematic reviews have not been able to establish an exact concordance and have expected the effects of the different treatment modalities to appear as soon as possible.[44] While others argue that there is indeed no significant relationship for the return of hearing. [44,45]

In addition to the above, it has been taken as a new hypothesis that the use of hyperbaric oxygen therapy is time-dependent, and its late administration therefore decreases its effectiveness.[44] In our results a mean of 8.8+/-19.8 weeks was highlighted, it is possible to analyse that the complete recovery was obtained in those patients who received the therapy in less than a month of evolution of the pathology, as time went by the effectiveness decreased notably, from the 14 weeks of onset of the symptomatology, being this a behaviour already documented previously. [44,46-48]

Hyperbaric oxygen as a rescue treatment is considered to have no effect after 6 months of evolution of the hypoacusis; its gain is limited after 3 months of evolution, where recovery is usually less than 5 dB.[49]

After analysing hearing improvement and recovery in the previous paragraphs, it is possible to conclude that patients with complete recovery had a hearing return of between 15 dB in relation to the contralateral ear (based on the classification used previously by Krajcovicova et al 2018), 8 of them also obtained changes in speech audiometry towards favourable perceptions (Table 10), coinciding with 100% auditory recognition in a range of 30 to 50 dB, almost reaching normality. These findings also coincide with the administration of hyperbaric oxygen therapy in a shorter time since the onset of the clinical picture, with a mean of 4 weeks (Table 6, figure 4). (Table 6, figure 4).

It is essential to highlight and consider such changes in speech audiometry as an extra for the analysis of this study, also with the aim of observing which patients may have useless or unusable hearing; this is why it has also been stipulated in the 2012 American Academy of Otolaryngology-Head and Nerck Surgery guidelines on idiopathic sudden hearing loss, that even subtle improvements in hearing in this area should be considered when selecting ears that are candidates for traditional hearing amplification. Specifically in the pathology described in this study, a WRS (Word recognition score) greater than or equal to 10 dB has been considered; our study shows patients who went on to improve in speech audiometry, an instrument used for understanding the spoken word, most of whose percentages were above 60% recognition, a fact that speaks of great possibilities for future hearing rehabilitation.[1]

Similarly, when correlated with pre-therapy treatments, patients with complete hearing recovery (26.3%) all received combined therapy for the return of hearing; 70% of them had received simultaneous therapy with systemic and intratympanic steroids and subsequently received hyperbaric oxygen therapy; while the remaining 30% received therapy with intratympanic steroids and then rescue treatment; the same data coincides with previous authors who claim the related use of therapies. [11,24, 40-43]

Therefore, hearing gains of at least 15 dB and favourable changes in speech audiometry improve social interaction and quality of life of patients in the long term, reducing long-term comorbidity, risks and psychological alterations. At the same time, it contributes to the possibilities of auditory rehabilitation.[1,4]

The impact of spontaneous recovery, however, is an important factor to consider in the breakdown of the effects of hyperbaric oxygen rescue therapy. So far, Mattox et al have reported a spontaneous return of hearing within 2 weeks of symptomatology onset in 29-78%[6], taking into consideration factors such as patient age, presence or absence of vertigo, degree of hearing loss and time between hearing loss and treatment. [6,50]

According to Rhee et al in their 2018 meta-analysis which included 16 non-randomised studies with a total of 2401 patients, the hearing gain with hyperbaric oxygen therapy is higher than with medical therapy at 15.6 dB. Also the mean in this study overall was a hearing gain of 15.3 dB (P 0.000). However, there remains a 38-65% chance of spontaneous improvement weeks after the onset of the condition. [51]

Similarly, Bennett et al in their systematic trial reported a 25% greater chance of hearing recovery in those who had hyperbaric oxygen therapy added to their treatment; this is supported by other authors such as Pezzoli and Ajduk, in the current study the chances of improvement were closely related when prior treatment with intratympanic and systemic steroids was given, with the percentage ranging from 70-78.5%. [20,22,52,53] Similarly, Yang et al, in their cohort study, reported a mean 22.5 dB PTA recovery after intratympanic and hyperbaric oxygen therapy, compared to a mean of 18.9 dB in the group where only intratympanic therapy was administered. [20,22,52, 53]

Underlying the combination of treatments is the vasodilator effect of hyperbaric oxygen on the organ of Corti and inner ear, especially the stria vascularis, which counteracts oxidative stress and vascular compromise, the main components of the hypothesised pathophysiology of idiopathic sudden sudden hearing loss, as well as the anti-inflammatory potential of intratympanic and systemic corticosteroids.[44]

Regarding the frequencies affected, a gain in voice frequencies predominated: 500, 250, 1000 and 6000 Hz, however the higher frequencies were more affected.before the start of therapy, 4000, 6000 and 8000 Hz, also reflected lower hearing gains compared to the low and middle frequencies, with a gain in dB above 10 dB with an overall range of 10±19.9 dB. [54,55] As an overall summary there was an improvement of more than 10 dB at all frequencies with a maximum standard deviation of 21.5 dB.[54,]Nakashima et al agree with other studies such as those by Topuz et al and Cho et al, that the tendency of hearing recovery is in the lower frequencies, giving good results at frequencies of 250, 500 and 1000 Hz; very close to the trends found in this research. Arguing that high frequencies tend to recover in a lower proportion in the general population. [47,54, 55]

Multiple investigations have concluded that the degree of hearing loss classified as profound (>91 dB) or >80 dB or at least above 61 dB, prior to hyperbaric oxygen therapy, has benefited the most from therapy. [56,57] This raises the question, whether hyperbaric oxygen therapy plays an important role for patients with idiopathic sudden sudden hearing loss who have a severe or profound degree of hearing loss. [54,56, 57]

The results focused on specific areas of hearing recovery and the repercussions on the quality of life that this entails for the patients; however, we did not want to leave aside the recovery and changes detected in the pre and post hyperbaric chamber speech audiometry, which have a great impact on this research; 57.8% improved their percentages of detection of spoken language in the diseased ear, a significant percentage in the communication and social interaction of patients with sudden idiopathic hearing loss. However, little literature has documented its importance and further research in this area is still essential.

Despite the treatment scheme used via oral, intratympanic or hyperbaric oxygen, there are also factors to which it is possible to attribute the prognosis and probability for the return of hearing. [7,10,35,36] The data collected took into account antecedents such as hypertension, type 2 diabetes mellitus, obesity and depression, with diabetes and hypertension predominating; other antecedents included smoking and alcoholism, and specific otorhinolaryngological factors such as acoustic trauma, contralateral congenital hypoacusis, etc.and Ramsay Hunt syndrome. It is important to highlight this history of multisystemic involvement, due to the impact on the microcirculation at multi-organ level and thus on the inner ear.[35]

Of the total who reported any comorbidity prior to therapy (14), 6 (15.7%) had several underlying comorbidities, and of these only 1 had full hearing recovery, compared to the remaining 8 (21%) patients with only one comorbidity, where 3 had full recovery.

A low percentage of hearing recovery has been documented when the clinical picture presents with vestibular symptomatology, with a flat audiometric pattern or morphologically described as a descending curve pattern, severe or profound hearing loss or poor speech audiometry results.[32-33]

Vertigo in turn comes into debate as a prognostic factor in hearing recovery, hypothesised to be related to ruptured membranes within the inner ear, in areas close to the vestibule, and as a factor that negatively interferes with the return of hearing. However, studies conclude that vertigo has little direct association with idiopathic sudden hearing loss, but affects hearing recovery through its interaction with the initial hearing level. [32,55]

The other factor involved in the evolution of hearing impairment is the type or degree of hearing impairment, where Wen et al. report poor recovery between 3.6% when the initial presentation of hearing loss is profound, however due to the characteristics of the research aimed at the efficacy of hyperbaric oxygen therapy, the percentages are not very comparable.[35]

In associations made by Capuano et al, no differences in hearing recovery were found in patients with smoking habits, diabetes and hypertension.[24] However, delays in recovery are reported in patients with hypercholesterolemia (>240 mg/dl), among other factors such as LDL and apolipoprotein B concentrations, likely responsible for triggering the pathogenesis of idiopathic sudden hearing loss.[24]

By way of summary, we can consider that despite the possible causes of sudden hearing loss, from vascular events, viral aetiology, among others, there are common characteristics in terms of pathophysiology in the inner ear, oxidative stress combined with a secondary vascular insufficiency and inflammatory process at cochlear level; we could then conclude that the perilymphatic oxygen tension decreases.[24] Cochlear activity requires an adequate blood supply, the organ of Corti and the stria vascularis are the most energy-demanding parts of the cochlea.[58] Therefore, oxygen supplied to regions where oedema and inflammation cause ischaemia, increasing intracochlear oxygen tension can decrease the oedema and reverse the ischaemia.[58]

Hyperbaric oxygen therapy is considered a safe treatment, with possible complications that do not cause major or long-term damage such as: barotrauma which has been reported in 9.2% and 0.04% per session, with women and children under 16 years of age at higher risk; others such as hypoglycaemia, dizziness, vertigo, anxiety attacks, dyspnoea, oxygen toxicity and chest pain. In general, the percentage of complications per session is reported to be 0.72%[44] and 17.4%, the possibility of presenting one or more complications. [38,39,44,59, 60]

In our investigation, tinnitus was the most frequent adverse event in 13.1% (5), 7.8% presented with dizziness or vertigo and one of them (2.6%) with barotrauma that manifested days after the end of treatment. [38,39,44,59, 60]

# XI. CONCLUSIONS

The results obtained in this research in terms of overall hearing gain in decibels and the subclassifications of hearing improvement and hearing recovery are very similar to those described in the existing literature, approximately 15 dB (p= 0.000).

The benefit of hyperbaric oxygen therapy was observed to be considerably greater when applied within an average period of 4 weeks from the onset of symptomatology, with efficacy decreasing over time and as the condition progressed.

It is also possible to conclude increased recovery at lower mid frequencies after therapy administration, beneficial changes in speech audiometry for speech perception and social interaction, and the possibility of improved clinical responses to combined therapies.

More research is needed on hyperbaric oxygen therapy, especially in conjunction with complementary studies of hearing and perception, speech understanding, quality of life and its use as both primary and rescue therapy, in order to standardise it.

# XII LIMITATIONS

1.-There were variations in the different treatments given to patients prior to hyperbaric oxygen therapy, which may have interfered with the results observed.

2.-The study was limited to a retrospective view, the validity of which is diminished. The study based its results on a classification of degree of improvement and recovery. However, the literature points out different ways of analysing it. 4.-Take into account the spontaneous recovery of hearing.

# XIII BIBLIOGRAPHY

Stachler RJ, Chandrasekhar SS, Archer SM, Rosenfeld RM, Schwartz SR, Barrs DM, et al. Clinical practice guideline: sudden hearing loss. Otolaryngol-Head Neck Surg Off J Am Acad Otolaryngol-Head Neck Surg 2012;146(3):1-35.

Krajcovicova Z, Melus V, Zigo R, Matisáková I, Vecera J, Kaslíková K. Efficacy of hyperbaric oxygen therapy as a supplementary therapy of sudden sensorineural hearing loss in the Slovak Republic. Undersea Hyperb Med 2018;45(3):363-70.

Dinç ASK, Çayönü M, Boynuegri S, Tuna EÜ, Ery1lmaz A, A KD, et al. Is Salvage Hyperbaric Oxygen Therapy Effective for Sudden Sensorineural Hearing Loss in Patients with Non-response to Corticostreoid Treatment? Cureus 2020;12(1):1-6.

4.-Kratochvílovà B, Profant O, Astl J, Holý R. Our experience in the treatment of idiopathic sensorineural hearing loss (ISNHL): Effect of combination therapy with HBO2 and vasodilator infusion therapy. Undersea Hyperb Med 2016;43(7):771-80.

Lawrence R, Thevasagayam R. Controversies in the management of sudden sensorineural hearing loss: an evidence-based review. Clin Otolaryngol 2015;40(3):176-82.

6.-Mattox DE, Simmons FB. Natural history of sudden sensorineural hearing loss. Ann Otol Rhinol Laryngol 1977;86:463-80.

7.-Eric R. Oliver, George T. Hashisalri. 160 Sudden Sensory Hearing Loss. In: Johnson J, Rosen C, Newlands S, Branstetter B, Casselbrant M, et al (Eds.). Bailey's Head and Neck Surgery-Otolaryngology. Lippincott Williams &. Wilkins, 5th Edition Philadelphia:Vol.2:2014: pp 2589-2596.

8.-Carneiro SN, Guerreiro DV, Cunha AM, Camacho ÓF, Aguiar IC. Hyperbaric oxygen therapy in sudden sensorineural hearing loss following spinal anesthesia: case reports. Undersea Hyperb Med 2016;43(2):153-9.

9.-Olex-Zarychta D. Successful treatment of sudden sensorineural hearing loss by means of pharmacotherapy combined with early hyperbaric oxygen therapy. Md journal 2017;96(51).

10.-Alexander Arts H. 150 Sensorineural Hearing Loss in Adults. In: Flint P, Francis H, Haughey B, Lesperance M, Lund V, Robbins K, et al. (Eds.) Cummings Otolaryngology-head And Neck Surgery. Elsevier Saunders. 6th Edition Philadelphia: Vol. III:2015:2331-5.

Chandrasekhar SS, Tsai Do BS, Schwartz SR, Bontempo LJ, Faucett EA, Finestone SA, et al. Clinical Practice Guideline: Sudden Hearing Loss (Update). Otolaryngol--head neck surg

2019;161(S1):1-45.

12.-Cadoni G, Cianfoni A, Agostino S, Scipione S, Tartaglione T, Galli J. Magnetic resonance imaging findings in sudden sensorineural hearing loss. J Otolaryngol 2006;35:310-316.

13.-Agrawal S, Sharma N. Complete recovery following hyperbaric oxygen therapy in idiopathic sudden sensorineural hearing loss--a report of two cases. Undersea Hyperb Med 2016;43(2):161-6.

Sharma A, Kirsch CFE, Aulino JM, Chakraborty S, Choudhri AS, Germano IM, et al. ACR appropriateness criteria hearing loss and/or vertigo. J Am Coll Radiol 2018;15(11s):321-331.

15.-Battaglia A, Lualhati A, Lin H, Burchette R, Cueva R. A prospective, multi-centered study of the treatment of idiopathic sudden sensorineural hearing loss with combination therapy versus high-dose prednisone alone: a 139 patient follow-up. Otol Neurotol 2014;35:1091-1098.

Hosokawa S, Hosokawa K, Takahashi G, Sugiyama K, Nakanishi H, Takebayashi S, et al. Hyperbaric Oxygen Therapy as Concurrent Treatment with Systemic Steroids for Idiopathic Sudden Sensorineural Hearing Loss: A Comparison of Three Different Steroid Treatments. Audiol Neurotol 2018;9;23:145-51.

Sevil E, Bercin S, Muderris T, Gul F, Kiris M. Comparison of two different steroid treatments with hyperbaric oxygen for idiopathic sudden sensorineural hearing loss. Eur Arch Otorhinolaryngol 2016;273(9):2419-26.

Suzuki H, Kawaguchi R, Wakasugi T, Do BH, Kitamura T, Ohbuchi T. Efficacy of Intratympanic Steroid on Idiopathic Sudden Sensorineural Hearing Loss: An Analysis of Cases With Negative Prognostic Factors. Am J Audiol 2019;28(2):308-14.

19.-Murphy-Lavoie H, Piper S, Moon RE, Legros T. Hyperbaric oxygen therapy for idiopathic sudden sensorineural hearing loss. Undersea Hyperb Med 2012;39(3):777-92.

Ajduk J, Ries M, Trotic R, Marinac I, Vlatka K, Bedekovié V. Hyperbaric Oxygen Therapy as Salvage Therapy for Sudden Sensorineural Hearing Loss. J Int Adv Otol 2017;13:61-4.

Gülüstan F, Yaz1c1 ZM, Alakhras WME, Erdur O, Acipayam H, Kufeciler L, et al. Intratympanic steroid injection and hyperbaric oxygen therapy for the treatment of refractory sudden hearing loss. Braz J Otorhinolaryngol 2018;84(1):28-33.

Pezzoli M, Magnano M, Maffi L, Pezzoli L, Marcato P, Orione M, et al. Hyperbaric oxygen therapy as salvage treatment for sudden sensorineural hearing loss: a prospective controlled study. Eur Arch Otorhinolaryngol 2015;272(7):1659-66.

23.-Rhee T-M, Hwang D, Lee J-S, Park J, Lee JM. Addition of Hyperbaric Oxygen Therapy vs Medical Therapy Alone for Idiopathic Sudden Sensorineural Hearing Loss: A Systematic Review and Meta-analysis. JAMA Otolaryngol Head Neck Surg 2018;144(12):1153-61.

Capuano L, Cavaliere M, Parente G, Damiano A, Pezzuti G, Lopardo D, et al. Hyperbaric oxygen for idiopathic sudden hearing loss: is the routine application helpful? Acta Oto-Laryngologica 2015;135(7):692-7.

25.-Almosnino G, Holm JR, Schwartz SR, Zeitler DM. The Role of Hyperbaric Oxygen as Salvage Therapy for Sudden Sensorineural Hearing Loss. Ann Otol Rhinol Laryngol 2018;127(10):672-6.

26.-Miao X, Xin Z. Different treatment protocols for moderate idiopathic sudden sensorineural hearing loss. Undersea Hyperb Med 2019;46(5):659-63.

27.-Almosnino G, Holm JR, Schwartz SR, Zeitler DM. The Role of Hyperbaric Oxygen as Salvage Therapy for Sudden Sensorineural Hearing Loss. Ann Otol Rhinol Laryngol 2018;127(10):672-6.

28.-Miao X, Xin Z. Different treatment protocols for moderate idiopathic sudden sensorineural hearing loss. Undersea Hyperb Med 2019;46(5):659-63.

29.-Kim SA, Ahn JH. Clinical Application of Hyperbaric Oxygen in Treatment of Idiopathic Sudden Sensorineural Hearing Loss. Korean J Otorhinolaryngol-Head Neck Surg 2016;59(7):490-4.

Hosokawa S, Sugiyama K-I, Takahashi G, Hashimoto Y-I, Hosokawa K, Takebayashi S, et al. Hyperbaric Oxygen Therapy as Adjuvant Treatment for Idiopathic Sudden Sensorineural Hearing Loss after Failure of Systemic Steroids. Audiol Neurootol 2017;22(1):9-14.

31.-Newman CW, Jacobson GP, Spitzer JB. Development of the Tinnitus Handicap Inventory. Arch Otolaryngol Head Neck Surg 1996;122:143-148.

Cho I, Lee H-M, Choi S-W, Kong S-K, Lee I-W, Goh E-K, et al. Comparison of Two Different Treatment Protocols Using Systemic and Intratympanic Steroids with and without Hyperbaric Oxygen Therapy in Patients with Severe to Profound Idiopathic Sudden Sensorineural Hearing Loss: A Randomized Controlled Trial. Audiol Neurootol 2018;23(4):199-207.

Ylldlrlm E, Murat Özcan K, Palall M, Cetin MA, Ensari S, Dere H. Prognostic effect of hyperbaric oxygen therapy starting time for sudden sensorineural hearing loss. Eur Arch Otorhinolaryngol 2015;272(1):23-8.

34.-Huafeng Y, Hongqin W, Wenna Z, Yuan L, Peng X. Clinical characteristics and prognosis of elderly patients with idiopathic sudden sensorineural hearing loss. Acta Otolaryngol 2019;139(10):866-9.

35.-Wen Y-H, Chen P-R, Wu H-P. Prognostic factors of profound idiopathic sudden sensorineural hearing loss. Eur Arch Otorhinolaryngol 2014;271(6):1423-9.

Choo O-S, Yang SM, Park HY, Lee JB, Jang JH, Choi SJ, et al. Differences in clinical characteristics and prognosis of sudden low- and high-frequency hearing loss. The Laryngoscope 2017;127(8):1878-84.

Ricciardiello F, Abate T, Pianese A, Mesolella M, Olivia F, Farrise P, et al. Sudden sensorineural hearing loss: role of hyperbaric oxygen therapy. Translational Med Rep. 2017;1:13-16.

38.- Weaver LK. Hyperbaric oxygen therapy indications. UHMS. 2008;12:215-218.

Hadanny A, Meir O, Bechor Y, Fishlev G, Bergan J, Efrati S. The safety of hyper- baric oxygen treatment-retrospective analysis in 2,334 patients. Undersea Hyperb Med. 2016;43(2):113-122

Li Y. Interventions in the management of blood viscosity for idiopathic sudden sensorineural hearing loss: a meta-analysis. J Health Resand Rev. 2017;4:50-61.

Li L, Ren J, Yin T, Liu W. Intratympanic dexamethasone perfusion versus injection for treatment of refractory sudden sensorineural hearing loss. Eur Arch Otorhinolaryngol. 2013; 270:861-867.

42.- Wu HP, Chou YF, Yu SH, Wang CP, Hsu CJ, Chen PR. Intratympanic steroid injections as a salvage treatment for sudden sensorineural hearing loss: a randomized, double-blind, placebo-controlled study. Otol Neurotol. 2011;32:774-779.

Zhou Y, Zheng H, Zhang Q, Campione PA. Early transtympa- nic steroid injection in patients with "poor prognosis" idiopathic sensorineural sudden hearing loss. ENT J Otorhinolaryngol Relat Spec. 2011;73:31-37.

Eryigit B, Ziylan F, Yaz F, Thomeer HGXM. The effectiveness of hyperbaric oxygen in patients with idiopathic sudden sensorineural hearing loss: a systematic review. Eur Arch Otorhinolaryngol 2018;275(12):2893-904.

Siegel LG. The treatment of idiopathic sudden sensorineural hearing loss. Otolaryngol Clin N Am 1975; 8:467-73.

Ceylan A, Celenk F, Kemaloglu YK, Bayazit YA, Göksu N, Ozbilen S. Impact of prognostic factors on recovery from sudden hearing loss. J Laryngol Otol 2007; 121:1035- 40.

Cho CS, Choi YJ. Prognostic factors in sudden sensorineural hearing loss: a retrospective study using interaction effects. Braz J Otorhinolaryngol 2013;79(4):466-470.

Edizer DT, Celebi O, Hamit B, Baki A, Yigit O. Recovery of idiopathic sudden sensorineural hearing loss. J Int Adv Otol 2015;11(2):122-126

Mathieu D, Marroni A, Kot J. Tenth European Consensus Conference on Hyperbaric Medicine: recommendations for accepted and non-accepted clinical indications and practice of hyperbaric oxygen treatment. Diving Hyperb Med. 2017;47:24-32.

50.- Rauch SD. Clinical practice. Idiopathic sudden sensorineu- ral hearing loss. N Engl J Med. 2008;359(8):833-840.

51.- Hara S, Kusunoki T, Honma H, Kidokoro Y, Ikeda K. Efficacy of the additional effect of hyperbaric oxygen therapy in combination of systemic steroid and prostaglandin E1 for idiopathic sudden sensorineural hearing loss. American Journal of Otolaryngology. 2020;41(2):1023-63.

Bennett MH, Kertesz T, Perleth M, Yeung P, Lehm JP. Hyperbaric oxygen for idiopathic sudden sensorineural hearing loss and tinnitus. Cochrane Database Syst Rev 2012;17(10):473-9.

Bennett M, Kertesz T, Yeung P. Hyperbaric oxygen therapy for idiopathic sudden sensorineural hearing loss and tinnitus: a systematic review of randomized controlled trials. J Laryngol Otol 2005;119:791-8.

54.- Topuz E, Yigit O, Cinar U, Seven H. Should hyperbaric oxygen be added to treatment in idiopathic sudden sensorineural hearing loss? Eur Arch Oto Rhino Laryngol 2003;

55.- Nakashima T, Yanagita N. Outcome of sudden deafness with and without vertigo. Laryngoscope. 1993;103(10):1145-9.

Fujimura T, Suzuki H, Shiomori T, Udaka T, Mori T (2007) Hyperbaric oxygen and steroid therapy for idiopathic sudden sen- sorineural hearing loss. Eur Arch Otorhinolaryngol 264(8):861-866.

Liu S, Kang B, Lee J, Lin Y, Huang K, Liu D et al. Comparison of therapeutic results in sudden sensorineural hearing loss with/without additional hyperbaric oxygen therapy: a retrospective review of 465 audiologically controlled cases. Clin Otolaryngol 36(2):121-128.

58.- Nagahara K, Fisch K, Yagi M. Perilymph oxygenation in sudden and progressive sensorineural hearing loss. Acta Otolaryngol 1983;96:57-69.

59.- Yang CH, Ko MT, Peng JP, Hwang CF. Zinc in the treatment of idiopathic sudden sensorineural hearing loss. Laryngoscope. 2011;121:617-621.

Yang CH, Wu RW, Hwang CF. Comparison of intratympanic steroid injection, hyperbaric oxygen and combination therapy in refractory sudden sensorineural hearing loss. Otol Neurotol. 2013;34:1411-1416.

# XIV ANNEXES

**Annex 1.** Products

This research work will generate a scientific article that will be published in a journal.
indexed.

**Annex 2.** Ethical aspects

The protocol was submitted to the Research Ethics Committee of the Centro de Investigación y Docencia en Ciencias de la Salud of the Universidad Autónoma de Sinaloa for evaluation and approval, in order to safeguard the dignity, rights and safety of those involved.

The World Medical Association's Declaration of Helsinki sets out ethical principles for medical research involving human subjects, and this Declaration is used and accepted worldwide. The principles set forth in this declaration are that physicians should promote and safeguard the health, welfare and rights of patients, including those who participate in medical research. It should be understood that the primary purpose of medical research involving human subjects is to understand the causes, course and effects of disease and to improve preventive, diagnostic and therapeutic interventions. All medical research must be subject to ethical standards that serve to promote and ensure respect for all human subjects and to protect their health and individual rights. The research project and method of study must always be described and justified in a research protocol. Research protocols should be submitted to an ethics committee prior to initiation of the study for consideration, comment, advice and approval. The privacy and confidentiality of the personal information of research participants must be safeguarded.

Within the Regulations of the General Health Law on research for health, the parameters under which medical research must be established are established. According to article 3, research for health includes the following development of actions that contribute to the knowledge of biological and psychological processes in human beings, knowledge of biological and psychological processes in human beings, knowledge of the links between the causes of disease, medical practice and social structure, prevention and control of health problems, knowledge and evaluation of the harmful effects of the environment on health. Article 13 states that research in which the human being is the subject of study must respect his or her dignity and protect his or her welfare and human rights. Article 16 states that the privacy of the individual research subject must be protected.

Under compliance with these statutes, this research seeks to safeguard the integrity, dignity, well-being and protection of rights of participants.


**Impact on the population participating in research**


The US incidence of idiopathic sudden hearing loss is 5-20 per 100,000 population and a total of 66,000 cases annually. The exact figure in the Mexican population remains unknown. This is why the present study will focus on the investigation of this pathology in Mexico.

This work will show the efficacy of hyperbaric oxygen therapy as a rescue treatment for the return of hearing, since this disease causes serious morbidity in the patient who suffers from it; it leads to disability of the individual in their daily life activities and compromises their quality of life by preventing adequate social interaction and communication, a problem that extends both in the short and long term. The aim is to improve the prognosis for hearing recovery and avoid any possibility of chronic damage and long-term disability.


**Scientific relevance in the design and conduct of the study**


Correct identification of such an emergency and timely treatment within the first few days of symptom onset is imperative, however, when more than two weeks have passed, the chances of hearing recovery diminish and therapeutic options are limited. An innovative option for rescue treatment is hyperbaric oxygen therapy, which has shown benefits in absolute hearing restoration of 5 to 12 dB, however, the dosage and frequency is still in the process of standardisation. It is for this reason that the present investigation focuses on the comparative hearing before and after treatment, and will contribute to the evidence of the efficacy of this therapy. However, the present study has its limitations, as the ideal design for testing the efficacy of a treatment is a retrospective study such as a clinical trial.

**Risk level**

Level I. No-risk research: This is a retrospective study that will use only data collection and clinical record review. There will be no intentional intervention or modification in the physiological, psychological and social variables of the individuals in the study.

**Benefits and risks**

This study includes patients with idiopathic sudden sudden hearing loss, undergoing rescue treatment with hyperbaric oxygen therapy sessions during the period from March 2020 to July 2023, treated at the Civil Hospital of Culiacán, regardless of their socioeconomic status or demographics, in order to contribute to the restoration of their hearing abilities, thus improving their social relationships, communication skills, coexistence and overall quality of life. It also aims to promote health and new evidence in the area and contribute to future research. Risks of the investigation concerning the handling of the information in the electronic file, for which all necessary measures will be taken to safeguard the personal data of those involved.

**Vulnerable population**

This study did not include a vulnerable population as it was a retrospective study with a review of clinical records.

**Confidentiality**

As stipulated in the General Health Law, according to Article 16, the privacy of the individual research subject will be protected in research involving human subjects. Personal data were stored in an Excel database, to which only the principal investigator had access. No personal data were disclosed at the time of publication of the results obtained.

**Conflict of interest**

There is no conflict of interest.No financial or other interests of benefit to the researcher or the institution are involved in carrying out this study.

**Annex 3**. Informed consent form with institutional seals: Not applicable.

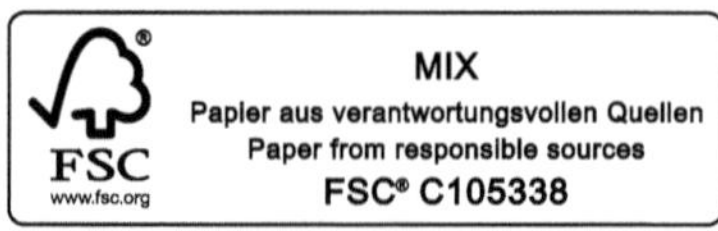

Printed by Books on Demand GmbH, Norderstedt / Germany